BEAT CANDIDA THROUGH DIET

A COMPLETE DIETARY PROGRAMME FOR SUFFERERS OF CANDIDIASIS

Gill Jacobs and
Joanna Kjaer

Vermilion
LONDON

13 15 17 19 20 18 16 14

First published in the United Kingdom in 1997 by Vermilion
an imprint of Ebury Press

This edition published 2001

Random House UK Limited Reg. No. 954009

Addresses for companies within the Random House Group
can be found at www.randomhouse.co.uk

A CIP catalogue record for this book is available from the British Library

The Random House Group Limited supports The Forest Stewardship Council
(FSC), the leading international forest certification organisation. All our titles that
are printed on Greenpeace approved FSC certified paper carry the FSC logo.
Our paper procurement policy can be found at www.rbooks.co.uk/environment

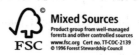

Mixed Sources
Product group from well-managed
forests and other controlled sources
www.fsc.org Cert no. TT-COC-2139
© 1996 Forest Stewardship Council
FSC

ISBN 978 0 09 181545 5

Typeset in Bembo and Gill Sans

Design & page make-up by Roger Walker/Graham Harmer

Printed and bound in the United Kingdom by
CPI Mackays, Chatham, ME5 8TD

Contents

Part III
The Beat Candida Diet Recipes

Acknowledgements

We would like to thank the following for their advice and help in the writing of this book:

Jane McWhirter for her thorough appreciation of all levels of candida control, from the dietary and practical, to the emotional and spiritual. Her commitment to not only the nitty gritty of how to get better, but also to a wider vision of change, has been, and continues to be, an inspiration to us both. Gillian Hamer for her hands-on experience in treating hundreds of cases a year. Her approach is a model of how to treat this condition, and is reflected in the team-work approach to candida of other therapists at All Hallows House, in the City of London. Dr John Briffa for his positive, but realistic, approach to recovery and change, his readiness to always listen, his skill as a communi-cator, and his understanding of the support that patients need. Joan Bullock, nutritional therapist and reflexologist, who takes the time to show her clients how to cook. Gwynne Davies, whose loss to this field through retirement is thankfully delayed by the books he will publish, and the Master Classes he will give. Dr Alan Hibberd for his constant reminders of the role of parasites in candida control, and the dangers of mercury amalgam fillings. Anya Harris for her perspective as an ex-sufferer, on the role of diet, and of stress in candida control, (and for permission to use her experiences as a case-study in this book). Antigoni Cogill-Ellis for her useful insights into how to run successful support groups, and how confused sufferers become with each new declaration of banned or permissible foods! All the participants in the Candida Workshops should also be thanked for increasing our understanding of the problems and pitfalls that inevitably occur during efforts to get well.

We also need to thank the team of experts connected to 'Kjaers Food for Life', who were always available at the end of the phone to answer some obscure question about the science of food, and how different manufacturing processes affected foods.

Finally, we would like to thank Joanna's daughter, George Brogden, for typing and practical support when it came to getting the recipes together, and all those, particularly Chris Thompsett and past customers at the 'Food For Life Restaurant', who tried out the results of Joanna's *Beat Candida Through Diet* recipes.

About the authors

Gill Jacobs

Gill Jacobs is author of *Beat Candida: From Thrush to Chronic Fatigue* (Vermilion, 1996), *Candida Albicans: Yeast and Your Health* (Optima 1990), and *The Natural Way: Chronic Fatigue Syndrome* (Element Books 1998).

A former sociology lecturer, and health education teacher, she became a health writer in order to publicise the plight of thousands of women and men who have problems with yeast infection and gut dysbiosis, and who find it hard to get help. For the past nine years she has been a trustee of the charity Action for ME and Chronic Fatigue, with a particular interest in nutritional approaches to recovery, and campaigning for wider recognition. Having run a series of one-day workshops for candida sufferers, as Candida Workshops, with the health writer Jane McWhirter, they now run conferences for holistic health practitioners. Together they have produced a three hour video on candida treatment and management, in order to provide support and encouragement to sufferers who are battling with their health.

Joanna Kjaer

Joanna Kjaer's cooking style has been influenced by her travels around the world. Her first major culinary venture was Joanna's Kitchen, making organic breads for the green markets at Spitalfields and Portobello in London.

Food for Life, the healthfood restaurant at the Hale Clinic opened soon afterwards. Here, with customer feedback, she was able to refine recipes, and learn more about food sensitivity from some of the leading practitioners in the field. In 1996 Kjaers Food for Life launched a range of organic breads, cakes and biscuits for special diets.

Joanna Kjaer continues to publish recipes while practising in Norfolk as a Dietary Therapist. She also works for Norfolk County Council Adult Education Health and Sports Studies.

Foreword

BY DR JOHN BRIFFA

When I first became interested in the subject of natural medicine I became aware of a good deal of information implicating candida albicans in a wide variety of conditions. From chronic fatigue to irritable bowel syndrome, and dandruff to insomnia, yeast was seemingly to blame. At medical school we were taught that candida was responsible for thrush in women, and would sometimes run riot in the bodies of the seriously ill. Now it was being suggested that this little yeast organism was an important factor in just about every illness for which the medical profession had no explanation. Naturally - bearing in mind what I had learnt during my medical training - I was sceptical.

However, my dealings with patients taught me that even when factors such as nutritional deficiencies and food sensitivity were corrected, a proportion of people did not get well. More out of desperation than anything else, I began to start treating selected patients with the anti-candida protocol. To my amazement, a diet low in yeast, sugar, alcohol and refined carbohydrates, supported with specific nutritional supplements brought about dramatic improvement in a great many of these patients. In a few, symptoms that had been around for 20 years or more vanished within a few days or weeks. My initial scepticism regarding the role of candida in modern day illness was quickly dispelled through my experience with patients.

Yet, while the anti-candida regime can often bring about near miraculous improvements in health for many people, no-one has ever claimed it was easy: the diet usually demands that individuals make sweeping changes to their diets and forego some of their favourite foods. Over the years I have become convinced that two factors are very important in determining an individual's success on the anti-candida regime. Firstly, they must understand the beast they are dealing with and why certain dietary changes are necessary. Secondly, the diet should be interesting, tasty and varied.

This book provides information that satisfies both these criteria. Gill has provided a clear account of candida, the problems it can cause and the principles behind its treatment. To complement this, Joanna has provided an array of mouth-watering recipes that will liberate those on an anti-candida regime from endless meals based around brown rice and vegetables. Together, Gill and Joanna make a formidable team. Follow the advise in this book and you can't fail to feel the benefit, both in terms of your health and your culinary repertoire.

Dr John Briffa BSc(Hons) MB BS(Lond)
Nutritional Physician
March 1997

Introduction:
The Diet Connection

The role of candida overgrowth in health and disease is not fully recognised by conventional medicine, despite the thousands of people who are undoubtedly affected by it, often as a result of over-use of antibiotics.

In fact there are thousands of scientific papers on the role of yeast and fungi in illness. Many are by veterinarians, or by doctors and medical researchers in Germany and Russia. Vets have to concern themselves with keeping animals alive and productive, and animals reared for food are exposed to the negative affects of constant antibiotic use. Both Germany and Russia are rye growing regions, where an appreciation of the natural 'souring' fermentation process is important because rye bread cannot be baked naturally. Thus microbiological research in this area developed out of commercial interests in the food and wine sector. The controversy and denials surrounding candida-related diseases in the USA and the UK are not so prevalent. German research on ME has investigated the role of candida overgrowth in the illness and found it to be present in a large proportion of cases.

The difficulty is that many who suffer from candida overgrowth do not know why they are ill or how to get better. And whilst conventional medicine in Britain and the USA is unwilling to take candida seriously, sufferers are forced to rely on self-help books such as this, media interest, and complementary medicine.

The importance of diet

When Jane McWhirter and I set up our first Candida Workshops we thought we knew what most people needed to get out of them – group support to give them renewed motivation, and hope. This was partly true. But equally the participants had a desperate and compelling need for inspiration and guidance on what and how to eat. The diet connection with candida seemed to be the biggest hurdle, and the biggest burden. Somehow, sufferers were stuck with the feeling of deprivation – and inadequacy. Whatever they had cooked before was no longer relevant. Omitting so many ingredients seemed a mammoth task. Finding the energy and time to manage new foods and new health principles was not easy, especially if cooking for others was part of the problem.

Our talks on the theory of candida overgrowth went down well, but the audience came alive and animated when Jane McWhirter assembled her temporary kitchen, and started to cook with infectious enthusiasm and creative inspiration. Then Joanna would wheel out her lunch and the workshop would positively hum with the sound of satisfied chatter as everyone experienced good food, which was organic, nutritious and sugar-, yeast- and wheat-free. We hoped that the positive experience of sharing food could be recreated in local support groups, where in addition, ideas could be exchanged, and motivation restored.

Clearly, there was a gap in the help that candida sufferers were getting. Practitioners were doing their bit – supervising the intake of probiotics, antifungals and nutritional supplements. Yet 'how' to prepare new food choices, after brief guidelines on what to avoid, was usually left to chance. One naturopath I spoke to groaned when I mentioned the subject of this book. His experience was that it was just too difficult to get people to change their eating habits. It was easier just to stick them on probiotics and hope for the best!

Traditionally, the anti-candida diet has come to be seen as

one which cuts out sugar, yeast and dairy products, with restricted fruit. A recommendation to cut out carbohydrates was reversed fairly quickly when some people starved themselves as well as the yeast. A survey of current diet books for candida still reveals a bewildering array of 'do's' and 'don'ts'.

Whilst everyone seems to agree that it is foolhardy to cut out complex carbohydrates, some books are wary about starchy carbohydrates, such as rice or potatoes, or vegetables with a high sugar content such as cooked carrots and squashes. Others take a hard-line view on fruit, banning it completely, until the yeast is under control.

After much confusion, and talking to practitioners and sufferers, we came to the conclusion that different approaches suit different people. In other words, there is no one way. Some books encourage 'going it alone', so that a strict diet replaces the need for supplements, although probiotics are usually included. Books with a wider food choice often place equal emphasis on the role of supplements and anti-fungals.

We hope that we have taken something from both approaches. By this we mean we have tried to incorporate some of the principles of food choice and health, whilst at the same time opting for a broad interpretation of what is permissible. The quality of the therapeutic relationship with the practitioner should never be underestimated as a factor to take into account here.

The *Beat Candida Diet* is not for life, and at some point it can gradually be replaced. But that does not mean that you should expect to be able to go back to old eating habits without a recurrence of your problems. We aim to provide you with tools for good health. These tools will equip you to make changes which will eventually become part of the way you react and relate to food choices. Hopefully, you will come instinctively to like what is good for you. That does not mean choosing foods because of food fads or fashions which try to dictate what is 'healthy'. It does mean that you will get to know what suits *your* body, and *your* metabolism.

A holistic view

The case-studies in this book demonstrate that the traditional answers from conventional medicine are not always relevant or helpful. Tests which come back negative, symptoms which are not connected, problems which are seen as 'normal' or 'psychological', sometimes lead us away from the real source of our problems. The answer for some of us is found in the gut.

As our lives become more and more hectic, as we allocate less and less time for the proper nourishment of our bodies and souls, as we demand and expect to be given 'magic pills' to do the work of our immune systems for us – so we push ourselves into chronic states of ill-health and fatigue. Taking control of your health today may be the best insurance for the future you can have.

Gill Jacobs, March 1997

The process of change

Spending some time to assess how to activate personal change is important, as you read through this book. The following factors need to be worked through, step-by-step, in order to trigger your personal commitment to overcoming your candida problem.

- The underlying reason for your current state of health and why change is needed must be clearly understood. It is not enough to rely on a practitioner to tell you. There may not be sufficient time for discussion, and you may not take in all the details during a consultation. You need to get to grips with how your body is reacting by reading and talking to others with similar experiences.
- There needs to be a personal recognition of the feelings which accompany deprivation when food is involved.
- When 'deprivation' is replaced by 'exchange' there is more possibility of moving on. This 'exchange' acknowledges the eventual benefits to be gained. The pay-off is being free of symptoms – and enjoying what you eat, especially when your range of choice is extended towards the end of the candida control programme.
- Try to rise to the challenge when you have to learn something new. Learn to tolerate the awkward phase of having to think

harder about what you are doing or choosing, rather than rely-
ing on old habits and quick responses.
- Giving yourself time is essential. It takes time to reorganise your
  kitchen, your shopping choices and your ways of cooking. You do
  not have to do everything all at once. You do not have to get it
  right straight away.
- Be prepared for toxic reactions as you move into the *Beat Candida Diet*. Remind yourself that this is part of the process of getting better. With the guidance of a practitioner you should be
  able to work out how to ease this transitional phase by getting
  nutritional support for your liver, taking time for more rest and
  sleep, or cutting back on antifungal treatments.
- We eventually learn to make the necessary changes our first pri-
  ority when we come to experience the inner value and long-
  term benefits. This means getting in touch with your body,
  listening to what it needs, and giving yourself the credit when it
  responds by getting better!
- Recognise that in order to make optimum health your first pri-
  ority you may need to give something else up temporarily, or
  negotiate with others to give you help. Keep in mind your ultimate goal of renewed energy from the candida control programme, and the *Beat Candida Diet*.
- Never underestimate the isolation of having this problem, and
  seek out sources of support to reinforce your resolve to get
  well. Do not, however, get sucked into situations which are negative. Support groups which provide an opportunity to 'moan'
  about symptoms could set you back, and chip away at your faith
  in your ability to get well.
- Progress is bound to be halted by periods of 'giving up' on the
  diet, or 'cheating'. This is natural. Keeping a food and symptom
  diary is essential to record how your body responds. A diary will
  also remind you how bad you were. Most recovered candida sufferers forget how many symptoms they had, unless they keep a
  record. Looking back reminds you how far you have come.
- Much depends on the reaction of family and friends, and your ability to defy the cynicism of others, who are threatened when their
  personal 'comfort zone' in food is challenged by alien and unfamil-
  iar choices. Try to include them in your attempts to understand
  how you got ill. If you are not successful, keep quiet, and wait to see
  if they are more receptive when your symptoms start to go.

Case histories

Debbie's Story

Debbie is 28 years-old with a responsible job in management. She works from 8am in the morning until 6pm or 7pm at night. She commutes for three and a half hours every day.

She had had the majority of her candida symptoms for four years before she stumbled across the diagnosis in a newspaper article. She had constant thrush, which was unrelieved by pessaries and Diflucan; constant sneezing for three or four hours every morning, persistent fatigue, with spaced out, dizzy feelings; itchy head; itchy throat; and muscle aches. For two years she could hardly stay awake in the afternoon, and would fall asleep in the evenings at 9pm, having slept on the train journey home. If she drank half a glass of alcohol she would have diarrhoea for a week, and develop mucous behind her nose and eyes. Bloating was constant, especially after bread, and eating caused pain. She was told by one specialist to cut out milk and fibre.

She also developed what her doctor finally diagnosed as Irritable Bowel Syndrome (IBS) alternating between constipation and diarrhoea. Advice from a nurse to get a book from a health food shop was the only help given. A smear test for the thrush finally came up with the result of 'candida overgrowth'. At this point she found a nutritionist to help her get better.

After four months of sticking fairly rigidly to the diet she has almost recovered. Her sneezing went after two weeks, her

thrush has cleared up, and she has 'heaps of energy'. All her
other symptoms have disappeared. Apart from the diet she took
Candicidin, Bio-Acidophilus, Vitamin C, GLA Complex, and
Replete. Her maintenance programme follows the advice on
page 112.

Of the diet she says:
'I didn't realise it would be quite so drastic. Luckily I had a few
days between my first consultation and the supplements arriv-
ing through the post. I cut out coffee, and read some books on
candida in that time, before starting on the diet. My nutritionist introduced me to a wonderful health food shop near my
work (until then I had relied heavily on supermarket ready
made meals) and I just asked the assistant to put in a basket anything that I could eat. Luckily she gave me a recipe for cashew
nut butter with vegetables and tahini sauce. It was delicious.

What made me do the diet and stick to it was the cost. My
supplements were very expensive. There seemed no point in
breaking the diet too often if I was paying all that money. I was
fairly scrupulous about keeping a food dairy and writing down
everything I ate. Then when I went back to my practitioner I
could show her and get her advice.

For breakfast I had orange walnut crunch with sheep's milk
in the week, and organic oats at the weekend. Now I am having
Ryvita with sugar-free jam. Nearly every day I had a jacket
potato, or a salad for lunch, with occasional Japanese take-away
sushis – the sea vegetables are a great help for candida.

The food diary was in the form of a spreadsheet, and I also
wrote down my feelings. At first I was scared to eat, and I got
very hungry, but I soon got into things, after reassurance from
my practitioner. To help with the hunger I carried round with
me toasted sunflower seeds.

In the evenings I usually eat stir-fry of vegetables, with loads
of ginger, lemon juice, garlic and onions, and soft goats cheese
added at the last minute. I also eat a lot of fish. I was lucky that
although my partner kept to his high meat diet, we always

shared the cooking, which meant that every other night I didn't have to cook. I don't know what I would have done without his support because sometimes I was too tired to cook and too tired to eat.

I am disturbed that I had to go all those years without any help, or knowledge about candida. I got better because I am stubborn, and I really wanted to get well. At first my mother was worried about my treatment, but now she wants to know more about the diet for herself. My view is that the diet is great to stick to for life. Obviously I want to expand it a bit. But I feel so well now. I could never go back to bread or sugar.'

Chris' Story

Chris is a thirty three year-old graphic designer, whose problems first started in 1993, although he had had a fungal infection on his back as a child, and a proneness to athlete's foot. He attended our Leeds Candida Workshop – one of only three men out of fifty women – at the start of his candida treatment in the autumn of 1996.

He developed a flu-like illness, which kept him off work for nearly a month, with extreme fatigue. He was given a two week course of antibiotics, after which he was left with an intense burning sensation on his scalp, and a feeling that his hair was being pulled. This lasted for the next three years, during which time he tried every conventional avenue to get help. His GP told him there was nothing wrong, and sent him away with no tests. A skin specialist could find nothing wrong, and a scalp specialist put him on a course of antibiotics, with steroids on his scalp. This made his symptoms worse.

In desperation he went to a health food shop and bought a book on fungal infections, and started to cut down sugar and yeast. But it was only when he read an article about someone whose life had been transformed by treatment for candida that he booked up an appointment with a nutritionist. Before he saw her he went back to his GP asking him to look through his notes for any reference to 'candida'. His GP confirmed that there was a note from the scalp specialist to say that there was 'very heavy candida under the scalp.'

'I was quite upset that nobody had told me. For all those years I was in such pain. And yet there it was in my notes all that time – a candida infection. My doctor denied negligence saying that I had been given antifungal tablets for a week – but no-one had told me what they were.'

Over the five months since he has received nutritional counselling his symptoms have significantly reduced. He was given Candicidin, probiotics, biotin, a multivitamin and mineral, and guidelines for the diet. Because he had already cut out bread, sugar and dairy products he found the transition relatively painless.

His main staples are rice, vegetables and fish, plenty of home-made soups, and vegetable curries. He tolerates cous cous, (wheat) and uses spelt flour. Lunches are easier because he now works from home.

His symptoms have gone away, to the point that he can now have a stressful day at work and not suffer with scalp pain. His hair stopped falling out after five months of the diet, and his stamina and digestive problems have improved. When he changed his antifungal to Candicidin he reacted with one bad day, which reminded him of how bad his symptoms used to be.

'It was good for me to get ill, in one sense. I have had to reassess everything. I changed my job which was quite stressful, with a lot of travelling, and now work from home. But it was not necessary for me to go through all that pain and distress. When are doctors going to realise the importance of diet, and nutrition, and the dangers of overusing steroids and antibiotics?'

Anya's Story

Anya is a professional healer in her mid-thirties, having changed direction from her first career as an associate director of a City bank. Four years ago, whilst still working in the City, she finally discovered that her many and varied symptoms were connected. She looks back on her twenties as a period in which she drove herself, in spite of having chronic fatigue, with numerous other symptoms. Her job was combined with an active social life, eating out five times a week. At work, her colleagues considered her to be an example to follow – she was careful with her diet, eating lots of pasta, she drank less then them, despite loving red wine, and she satisfied her craving for sugary drinks by drinking 'only' Diet Coke. She took aerobics so seriously that she trained to be an instructor. Despite being ill she looked well. Her will and her 'driven spirit' kept her going.

Her best time of day was between waking up and eating breakfast. She would have tea with sugar and toast and marmite, and from that point went down hill. The cramps from eating were only eased by more eating, so that an hour later she had to have more food, often chocolate bars at work, to satisfy her constant sugar and yeast cravings. Finally she realised that she she felt less pain if she didn't eat.

'Every time I ate I felt uncomfortable. As soon as I realised I didn't want to eat I knew had a problem. I was having supper with a friend and when she offered me bread I declined, saying that it hurt. When I mentioned that I also had thrush, she handed me Leon Chaitow's book on candida. I filled in the questionnaire and found I had thirty symptoms.'

Among them were sinus problems, dry skin, permanently sore eyes, hives, sore throats, fatigue, frequent urination, bloating, cramps, digestive problems, sugar cravings, PMT, painful periods. The list was endless. She immediately put herself on a yeast- and sugar-free diet with the result that after a week she found she was still awake at 10pm at night. It felt so strange she remembers ringing her friends to let them know.

Her first action was to take herself to her GP, letting him know her response to eliminating yeast and sugar. He said that candida was a fashionable diagnosis for the upwardly mobile, and that it was pure coincidence that she was better on the diet. Anya was determined not to let this go. She handed him the book, and told him to read it and her notes, saying that she would come back a week later. At the next meeting he agreed with her diagnosis, and offered her anti-fungal drugs. She declined, finding a nutritional therapist to help her instead. Seven months later when she went back to her GP 'heaps better', to let him know for the sake of others behind her, he was not interested.

During that seven months she had to learn to cook, and to read labels for the first time. Her first task was to get into the routine of shopping for the new foods. She kept her cooking very simple, but experimented with different quiches using non-wheat flours and sheep's milk. Because she was always hungry, she made biscuits to carry round with her. She lived mainly on tuna omelettes with fresh greens, and brown rice with vegetables. She learnt to roast peppers, grill courgettes, and use aubergines. Her best discovery was the convenience and speed of cooking fresh fish.

The detoxification phase in the early stages of the diet and control programme was very difficult to cope with, because she came off coffee at the same time. Her symptoms were worse than before, and she ached all over, developed acne, headaches, and bad breath. Throughout she continued to work. It was at this stage that she felt she needed support. She was living on her own, her colleagues were unaware of what she was going through, and her friends did not understand. Together with Jane McWhirter she started the All Hallows Candida Support Group in the City of London.

Every now and then she would break the diet, which she found very unsociable. (At one point her food intolerances were so extreme she had to give up all grains.) But she would always regret eating the wrong foods, although as she moved towards getting better, each recovery time reduced from a week to a couple of days. Throughout she was seeing an experienced practitioner who put her on supplements, natural anti-fungals and probiotics, and gave her dietary advice.

Assessing her recovery, Anya admits that she is now glad she became so ill. She knows that if she had carried on, without taking responsibility for her health, she would have either developed ME or had a breakdown. One of the most important lessons she was to learn was that diet alone was not enough. She had to sort out the stresses in her life as well.

'Being ill made me take stock, and educate myself about a lot of things. There was no way I was going to get better in my work environment. I took responsibility, saw a different way of life where I didn't need to struggle, and gave up my well-paid job because my health was more important. Rest is one of the biggest healers, and I wasn't getting any whilst working in such a stressful job. I was very fortunate to have enough savings to take this drastic step! Although I am hard-up now its been worth it'

Her recovery was not completed without three additional factors coming into play. She worked on herself emotionally, she had acupuncture to sort out blocked energies, and she had her mercury fillings removed. Although her candida symptoms went, her food intolerances suddenly increased. A kinesiologist alerted her to the need to remove the mercury, and from that point her health permanently improved. With a few child-bearing years left, she is relieved that she escaped having the hysterectomy. Since the candida treatment her periods are regular, painless, and trouble-free. Anya is sad that so many think that because tiredness is common it is normal. Now, her energy no longer needs to be 'driven' – it is fully charged and supported by a healthy body.

Part I
The Candida Problem

Chapter One

Candida explained

Is candida your problem?

Do you suffer from a bloated stomach, sugar cravings, fatigue, thrush, sore throat, digestive disturbances, wind, anal itching, PMT, cystitis, hormonal irregularities, food intolerances, skin problems, alcohol intolerance, bad breath, nail infections, mood swings, unexplained muscle pain or aches in the joints, weight fluctuations and 'foggy brain'?

If you have some of the above symptoms, there is a strong possibility that you have an imbalance of gut bacteria caused mainly by the overuse of antibiotics, a diet which encourages fermentation, and underlying stress. This is popularly known as *candida* or *candidiasis*.

Are you continually visiting the doctor without getting to the bottom of what is wrong? Are you at your wits end with a hyperactive child? Do you think that because you are a man yeast infections do not apply to you? Do you associate thrush only with vaginal infections? Do you think that feeling tired all the time or living with recurrent thrush and cystitis, is normal?

Everyone, regardless of sex or age, can be affected by problems of yeast or fungal overgrowth. Babies can be born with thrush in the mouth, picked up from the vaginal passage during birth. Children can be hyperactive because of candida over-

growth. Men can develop fungal skin problems, alcohol intolerance, bloating, anal itching, irritability and mood swings.
Candida should be investigated as the linking cause. Women
need not tolerate chronic ill health. It is not normal to be tired
all the time, and the numerous causes should always be investigated. Candida is likely to be involved if there is persistent
thrush and cystitis. (See page 51 for a symptom questionnaire.)

Is candida connected to other illnesses?

Other conditions which are thought, or suspected, to have a
candida connection are as follows:

- myalgic encephalomyelitis (ME) or chronic fatigue syndrome (CFS)
- endometriosis
- allergies
- fibromyalgia
- infertility
- diabetes
- irritable bowel syndrome (IBS)
- heart disease
- auto-immune diseases (lupus, thryroiditis, colitis, Crohn's
  disease, multiple sclerosis and rheumatoid arthritis)
- allergic conditions (hay fever, asthma, psoriasis and eczema)
- AIDS

The list is long. But there are enough cases of improvement and
recovery with antifungal treatment and diet to warrant more
than a suspicion that candida or fungal overgrowth is pervasive
and central to many twentieth century diseases. But thousands
remain oblivious to the role of nutrition and diet, and the
importance of intestinal health. This is not for a lack of con-
vincing scientific research. The association between scurvy and
vitamin C deficiency was originally treated with scepticism
and was finally scientifically proven years after it had been
common knowledge that lemon juice could keep scurvy at bay.

In time, the association between yeasts, moulds, fungi and health too will eventually be accepted - but only after a great deal of further confusion and chronic, avoidable, ill-health.

Terminology

Candida is a yeast mould, with different strains and types, the most pervasive being *candida albicans*. Other microbes which cause problems are harmful bacteria, such as E coli (as opposed to the usually more predominant beneficial bacteria), parasites and amoeba. A more accurate term would be *gut dysbiosis* because that takes account of microorganisms in the digestive tract other than just candida.

Dysbiosis means a state of disordered microbial balance which causes disease. In America they are starting to use the short-hand term GDS, or Gut Dysbiosis Syndrome. Throughout this book we will use the term *candida*, whilst acknowledging the value of eventual acceptance of the more accurate term gut dysbiosis. Another term in use in America is Candida Related Complex (CRC). This takes account of the fact that each person experiences candida in a different way, with a different constellation of symptoms.

What does candida overgrowth do?

Yeasts, of which candida is one, are single celled organisms which are part of the general family of moulds. As such they are similar to the moulds which grow on bread or mushrooms, or which colonise food when it is no longer fresh, causing it to ferment and decay. They are useful because they alert us to old food which is 'past its sell-by date' and which is no longer nutritious and life-giving. When they live on or inside humans we need to be aware of their potential for toxic harm, when allowed to get out of hand. Their role, even when kept in balance, is not beneficial, and as such they should be seen as parasites, living off a host – in this case a human one.

Candida is usually harmless when kept under control in a healthy body. It lives on the skin and on any mucosal surface – the throat and nose, the vagina and in the gut. The gut is usually the initial source of colonisation, although there can be localised sources of skin infection, such as dandruff or ringworm. Candida and other fungi produce a large number of biologically active substances called mycotoxins. The function of these toxins is to protect fungi from viruses, bacteria, parasites, insects, animals and humans.

The beneficial flora, co-residents of the digestive tract, are predominantly lactobacilli and bifido bacteria. They help to regulate digestion and absorption of food. They also act as gatekeepers, defending us from harmful pathogens, and keeping the colonies of yeasts in check. Other partners in the struggle for control are an efficient immune system and the correct level of acidity in our guts, referred to as the pH level.

With the right conditions candida can seize the opportunity and multiply, in the same way that yeast rises with sugar in breadmaking. It feeds on undigested sugars and starch, and changes form from a yeast to a fungus.

Thus there are two kinds of yeast to take account of, the second of which develops and grows out of the first in the right conditions:

- the commensal, benign yeast which causes mild overgrowth, because it is confined to living on fecal waste, encouraged by undigested food and low beneficial bacteria.
- the mycelial fungal form, which develops hyphae, or long filaments. It can produce gases and waste products, and sometimes alcohol. 'Leaky gut' can result when it uses its roots to penetrate through the mucosal barriers and into the tissues. This allows toxins, ie. poisonous waste products, to gain access to the blood stream, along with large food molecules which are incompletely digested. The immune system is triggered into action, causing inflammation, excess mucous production, and many of the symptoms associated with can-

dida, such as food intolerance, fatigue, hormonal irregularities, headaches and arthritis. If the immune system is overloaded in this way, and compromised by stress, it fails to meet the challenge, and yeast problems persist.

The problem is that once this vicious cycle kicks in it is hard to stop more and more symptoms and reactions. This is because the liver, the organ most responsible for handling waste products from the bloodstream, becomes overworked and congested. At the same time, as more and more inflammation occurs in the intestines in response to the problem, the normal process of digestion is sabotaged even further.

This applies particularly to the final process in the breakdown of starchy carbohydrates and complex sugars. This involves the membranes of cells lining the intestinal tract, and the minute projections called microvilli, at the point where foods are finally assimilated into the bloodstream. (The simple sugar, glucose, requires no digestion and is usually absorbed by the cells of the small intestine.) Villi flattened by excessive mucosal production in an irritated gut, will fail to complete the process of digestion. Undigested starches and sugars result, producing a ready source of food for fungal activity.

Elaine Gottschall, in her fascinating account of how she cured her daughter's ulcerative colitis through a diet of restricted carbohydrates which she followed for seven years, shows how undigested, unabsorbed carbohydrates remaining in the intestine can serve as 'the soil of the body' which encourage the growth of microorgnisms, such as bacteria and candida. (*Breaking The Vicious Cycle: Intestinal Health Through Diet.*) Her diet also helps Crohn's disease, and coeliac disease. She shows, using scientific studies, how the villi are able to recover when the offending foods, such as sucrose, starch and lactose, are removed from the diet. Her diet restricts carbohydrates more than is necessary for candida control however and there is other research to suggest that restricting carbohydrates without antifungal therapy can cause the candida to move deeper within tissue layers. It can adjust its metabolism from carbohydrate to protein, producing enzymes which digest protein, at the same time changing into the mycelial (fungal) form. 'Thus fungi become tissue invasive as they go foraging for new sources of food' (*Candida and Gut Dysbiosis Information Foundation Newsletter*, January, Vol. 2, No. 2, page 1, summarising untranslated German research.)

Candida and parasites

Candidiasis may be playing an important role in increasing the capability of various gut parasites to cause harm. Dr Alan Hibberd's clinical observations suggest that gut protozoal and *blastocystis hominis* infections are frequently found in gut candidiasis sufferers, and play an important part in symptoms which are attributed to candida. Dr Hibberd, a clinical ecologist and clinical toxicologist, states that approximately 50 percent of longstanding candida cases in the UK are complicated by one or more of the following parasites: *giardia lamblia, dientamoeba fragilis, endolimax nana, cryptosporidium parvum, entamoeba histolytica, chlostridium difficile*, and *blastocystis hominis*. ('Gut Parasitic Infections', *BioMed Newsletter*, No 9.) An awareness of parasitic activity should form part of candida control programmes.

Causes of candida overgrowth and symptoms

We all have candida living inside us. However, there need to be additional factors which cause the number of yeasts to increase to such an extent that they threaten our health. The list is as follows:

● antibiotic use
● the birth control pill
● Hormone Replacement Therapy
● steroids
● immuno-suppresive drugs and weakened immunity

- a diet high in refined carbohydrates and sugar
- prolonged stress
- heredity
- lack or insufficiency of hydrochloric acid in the stomach
- pancreatic enzyme deficiency

Antibiotics

Antibiotics are taken to kill harmful bacteria but they cannot distinguish between friend and foe, and kill beneficial bacteria at the same time. If you take repeated courses of antibiotics you are at risk of creating yeast problems, because there will not be enough beneficial bacteria, to keep the yeast in check.

Around 100,000 women in the UK each year take four or more courses of antibiotics for persistent cystitis. They are not always told by their doctors of the possible side-effects as a result of this. When they start to develop signs of candida overgrowth, such as persistent thrush, they are often unaware that the cause may be antibiotics. A change of diet, as outlined in this book, and nutritional support, will often prevent future bladder infections as well as all the other symptoms. Meanwhile, thousands of other women are unaware of the dangers, and the cycle is repeated.

If we take the attitude that we need not care about our health until we are ill, because we can be 'cured' by antibiotics, we fail to realise the importance of taking responsibility for our own health or the possibilities of preventing illness by the way we look after ourselves, and the way we nourish ourselves. By nurturing our immune system, our natural ability to fight infections, we can ensure that antibiotics are reserved for the times when they are really needed.

Each year world antibiotic production increases by 5 percent. In the USA alone 160 million prescriptions for antibiotics were written in 1995. Exposure to antibiotics is also unavoidable when we eat meat which is intensively reared. Factory farming could not survive without antibiotics.

A newspaper article in Britain (*The Observer*, 8 December 1996) quoted Professor Stuart Levy, director of the Centre of Drug Resistance at Tufts University, Boston, saying that society is facing one of its gravest public health problems – the emergence of infectious bacteria with resistance to many, and in some cases all, available antibiotics. Fourteen thousand Americans die each year from infections with drug-resistant bacteria that they picked up from hospital.

Antibiotics, thought to be our lifesavers, are now, as a result of abuse by overuse, one of the largest threats to health there is. A prominent critic of the overuse of antibiotics is Professor Richard Lacey, a medical microbiologist. In his clinic at Leeds University he finds that of all the people who have had their infection identified in his laboratory, less than one in 100 has been treated appropriately with antibiotics. Moreover, most of the infections are self-limiting, in that they will clear up eventually by themselves without any use of drugs. This has been confirmed by recent research at the University of Southampton, which shows that hot drinks of lemon and honey, or a similar remedy, will ease a sore throat as quickly as a course of antibiotics. The conclusion that antibiotics should be avoided by doctors in all but severe illnesses is confirmed by this research. It also confirms that antibiotics increase the risk of further infection by altering the bacteria in the throat, and limiting the development of natural immunity. (Reported in *The Times*, 7 March 1997.)

Another example of the increasing use of antibiotics in the UK is over-prescription for middle ear inflammation in children. Around one in five children under the age of four experience this problem every year – most will be prescribed antibiotics. Yet one cause of earache is often the excess mucous production that comes with the predominance of dairy products in our diets. Without understanding this, many parents are unable to take their children off the antibiotic treadmill. Children then become prime candidates for yeast overgrowth at a stage when their defences against it are still being developed.

The birth control pill and hormone replcement therapy

There is an association between candida and hormone levels, in that candida thrives on progesterone, found in the pill and hormone replacement therapy (HRT), and steroids. This is one reason why most women prone to thrush get more problems in the week before their periods when progesterone levels are high. The birth control pill also causes nutritional deficiencies which affect the mucous membranes and their ability to defend against fungal penetration. Sometimes the very problems for which women are prescribed HRT have been caused by candida overgrowth.

Steroids

Steroids form part of the following drugs: Prodnisolone, Hydrocortisone, inhalers such as Beconaze and Becotide, and creams such as Betnovate. Steroids are hormones which are naturally produced in the body, as part of the immune response. When given in drug form in larger amounts than can be produced naturally they act to suppress our own immune system, and destroy the delicate balance of micro-ecology. Thus, although they may keep down the symptoms whilst they are being taken, they can trigger problems as a result of yeast overgrowth, and other distressing side-effects. Steroids can be life-saving in certain situations and withdrawal from then should always be gradual and under medical supervision. However, where possible, natural alternatives should always be considered.

Immuno-suppressive drugs and weakened immunity

Chemotherapy dismantles our immune response, and our ability to defend against fungal invasion. In fact, doctors are familiar with candida problems as a side-effect of chemotherapy, because its occurence in these cases is so extreme that candida becomes visible and unavoidable. Thus cancer patients may die of complications caused when lungs are invaded by fungal overgrowth, rather than necessarily the cancer itself.

In AIDS patients the immune system is so weak that candida can cause general blood poisoning. One of the most visible symptoms of early AIDS is thrush in the mouth. This is confirmation that there is a fungal problem lower down the digestive tract, which has become chronic enough to travel upwards to the throat and beyond. Just treating thrush in the mouth will not, therefore, prevent the problem recurring.

Bottle feeding

Ninety percent of our *Bifido* bacteria is established in the first two days of life via colostrum and breast milk. Missing out on this boost for the ecology of our digestive tract *may* lead to problems later on. Bottle feeding, if it is combined with high sugar drinks and sugary foods during early childhood, can be an unfortunate combination because without adequate Bifido protection, candida can be encouraged to take hold, leading to problems of hyperactivity, and food sensitivity.

Sugar

Whilst it is true to say that we are what we eat, it is even truer to say that we are what we absorb. The problem for many is that we are bombarded with conflicting messages about what is, and what is not, a healthy diet. There is general agreement however that a high sugar diet, with refined carbohydrates (e.g. white flour) can predispose you to candida. See page 1 for a more detailed discussion of the diet connection.

Stress

It is a myth that experiencing stress is an entirely negative experience. Many of us are stimulated and energised by a healthy level of stress. It only becomes negative when we feel we are limited in our choices, or are unable to combine action with rest and relaxation. For women, stress is often about balancing personal needs with competing demands.

Scientists who have studied the relationship between stress and the body agree that stress has physical effects as well as emotional ones. Some studies (Kiecolt–Glaser et al, 'Psychosciaal modifiers of immunocompetence in medical students', *Psychosomatic Medicine* 46: 7–14, 1984) even go so far as to say that there is no chronic disease without chronic stress preceding it.

It is hard to motivate ourselves to change old patterns and habits. It is only when we become ill and have a problem with recovery that we are forced to take stock and work out how we may have contributed to the problem. It seems that only when some of the physical symptoms are reduced, through nutrition and diet, can enough energy be found to tackle other contributing causes, such as stress.

Candida and heredity

Our external features are determined by our inherited genes. So too is the health of our immune system. Heredity may be a factor in candida–related problems. Often our 'constitution' is as important a factor in determining how we respond to stress, as the environment or our state of mind. This does not mean that there is nothing to be done to avoid getting ill, or getting better. There are many other factors which contribute to wellness which are under our control.

Hydrochloric acid and pancreatic enzyme deficiency

If the acidity and activity of the gastric juices in the stomach are too low:

1. Putrefactive bacteria and yeasts, taken in with food, can start to grow.

2. Passed onto the the small intestine this mass of poorly
   digested fermenting food overwhelms the system, leading to
   depleted digestive enzymes.
3. This causes excess mucous production and diarrhoea.
4. Allergies are often the end result.

Pancreatic enzymes such a protease, lipase, and amylase, help
digest and destroy fungi found in food. Supplements can be
taken to boost enzyme levels and increase stomach acid, and
tests are available to accurately assess whether they are needed
(see chapter 4.).

Why is candida not recognised by conventional medicine?

Intestinal disorders are increasing, and include, apart from candida overgrowth, other conditions, such as Irritable Bowel
Syndrome (IBS), Coeliac's disease, and Crohn's disease.

Conditions that can be neatly defined have come under the
wing of scientific medicine, others, such as candidiasis, have
slipped through the net of credibility. Conventional medicine
has been forced to take notice in situations of severe weight
loss, or when the related symptoms seem confined to the
bowel. Sometimes, when drugs do not work, the medical profession has looked to the sufferer's mental state for a cause of
illness. It has been able to ignore candida overgrowth as a
factor because symptoms are wide-ranging and often found
throughout the body, and they are not traditionally perceived
as being connected to a single cause. Until recently tests for
candida overgrowth have been unavailable or unreliable.

How long has candidiasis been known about?

Candidiasis was first brought to light in the USA in 1977 by a
doctor, Dr Orian Truss, and then subsequently popularised and

publicised by the books of another doctor, Dr William Crook. In fact, the role of gut dysbiosis and diet had been highlighted some years before by a minority of physicians who became convinced that diet was the only way to cure problems of wasting, diarrhoea and digestion. Elaine Gotschall quotes evidence that in 1904, coeliac children were found to have stools with abnormally large numbers of fermentative and putrefactive bacteria, suggesting a dietary link, allowed to take hold without the normal control exerted by beneficial bacteria. In the 1940s Dr Josef Issels, a leading cancer specialist who advocated the role of nutrition in cancer care, wrote about the importance of balance in the ecology of the gastrointestinal tract. He warned that an imbalance with candida growth was one of the possible causes of cancer.

However, the growth of antibiotics from the late 1940s onwards, and our reliance on them to 'cure' bacterial infection, swept aside a minority awareness of the role of diet in health and disease. Why, when you could take a pill and lose your symptoms within days, bother with longer term cures? The fact that one course of antibiotics might not be enough, because infections and symptoms returned, was no matter. We took what we were given, and later demanded, and got on with our lives. Until, that is, the consequences of our actions started to rebound.

The next chapters look in more detail at the consequences of candida overgrowth, and how to test for and diagnose whether you have this problem.

Chapter Two

How we digest food

Digestion

Having read about what candida is, and the problems it can cause, it may also help to understand a little about how we digest food. So much of the process of eating is done without thinking of the consequences of what and how we eat. Whilst some of the following technical details may seem complex at first, you will soon become familiar with the basic facts. Without a 'magic pill' you are going to have to get to know how your body works as the first step in reversing old habits and choices.

Digestion is the process which breaks down food into substances that can be absorbed and used by the body for energy, growth and repair. The digestive system depends on a number of different organs, glands and their enzymes to enable this process to take place.

What is the gut?

The gut refers to the inside of the gastrointestinal tract. It is a highly specialised, elongated muscular tube whose function is to break down food and to extract the nutrients. Whatever is left over is deposited as waste. It is technically outside the body, because it is open to exposure at both ends, via the mouth and the anus.

What happens in the gut is normally beyond our conscious awareness, provided everything functions as it should. When we talk about a 'gut feeling' we are referring to something deep and

pH scale

The body is naturally alkaline, and the pH (the balance between acid and alkaline) of the bodily fluids, including the blood, should be 7.4, which is slightly alkaline. If your pH veers more towards acidity, through stress or an acid forming diet, it will allow yeasts, viruses, parasites and cancer cells to thrive. When the body becomes acidic, it has a hard time ridding itself of the resultant acid wastes. The stored reserves of alkaline minerals become depleted. They are sodium, calcium, potassium and magnesium. We will be looking at which kinds of foods are alkaline-forming in Chapter 7. The ideal is to eat in a balanced way so that acid-forming foods form a much lower percentage of food on your plate than alkaline ones.

If your body is too acidic less oxygen is available to the cells, leading to fatigue and lack of mental agility.

instinctive, which we do not analyse too much but take on trust. When something goes wrong in our gut, as with candida overgrowth, we can no longer rely on unconscious processes. We have to unravel the process in order to intervene and put things right.

The gut has three main components. They are the lining, referred to as the mucosa, the muscles and the digestive glands, such as the pancreas and the liver. The breakdown of the large molecules of food is achieved by enzymes. These are produced by the organs attached to the gut, and they are responsible for many of the chemical reactions involved in digestion. Some enzymes break down protein, some break down different kinds of carbohydrates, and other break down fats.

Enzymes require ideal conditions in order to do their job effectively. They operate best at body temperature, and at particular levels of acidity and alkalinity.

The process of digestion

Digestion starts in the mouth, where chewing breaks up the food, and stimulates the production of saliva which starts the breakdown of starchy foods. Well moistened, the food can then be swallowed.

In the stomach a mixture of chemicals is produced: mucous, hydrochloric acid and the protein-digesting enzyme, pepsin. Mucous protects the stomach lining from being damaged by the acid, which is needed to break the proteins into peptides. The high acidity also kills off any putrifying bacteria which may have gained entry with food. Stomach upsets occur when there is insufficient acid or pepsin, leading to fermentation if yeasts or other micro-organisms are present. It is interesting that we all vary in the amount of acid and pepsin we produce, and the amount that we need.

With much churning, the food is eventually passed on to the first part of the small intestine, called the duodenum. The food by this stage should be a thickish, acidic liquid. It is called chyme. It is now exposed to the majority of digestive enzymes from the pancreas, and the lining of the duodenum. Bile is produced from the liver, and is transported via the gallbladder, for the digestion of fats. At this stage the juices become alkaline in order to neutralise the acidic, partially-digested chyme. The enzymes here work best in an environment which is slightly alkaline or neutral.

Until now not many nutrients have been absorbed, but as the food and digestive enzymes interact in the small intestine more and more nutrients are absorbed through the lining of the gut wall into the bloodstream.

The digested food then enters the jejunum and ileum, further down the small intestine, where the final stages of chemical change takes place. Most food absorption takes place in the ileum which contains millions of minute projections called villi on its inner wall. Glycerol, fatty acids and dissolved vitamins are carried through into the lymphatic system, and poured out into the bloodstream. The lymphatic system is a secondary circulation system that carries fats to cells, collects and filters fluid from tissues through the lymph nodes, and is a central feature in the activity of the body's immune system.

Stress and digestion

The immune system is the body's defence against infection. If you are healthy, your immune system is constantly on the alert to ward off anything which might hurt or harm you. One of the factors which contributes to weakened immunity is stress, and this is most clearly demonstrated in our digestive tract. Mucosal cover of the lining of the digestive tract prevents dehydration, and invasion. Thus one of our main defences is mucosal exclusion. This barrier can become weakened when we are unhappy or stressed.

- Secretory IgA is part of the body's immune protection in the mucosal lining of the gut. It is an anti-inflammatory protein molecule capable of trapping invading bacteria. It is protected from enzyme activity, whose job it is to digest other proteins for absorption through the gut wall. The colon produces more secretory IgA(90%) than other areas. We produce a minimum of 3 gramms, and up to 7 gramms, a day.

- The steroid hormone cortisol, raised by stress, subdues the immune system, and the most susceptible to its action is mucosal immunity, mostly in the form of secretory IgA. Secretory IgA was shown to be reduced in one American study when students prepared for and took exams. It took three weeks to return to normal. Dr Ilyia Elias is Director of the Diagnos-Techs Laboratory in Washington State, USA, one of the leading centres for testing gut dysbiosis and adrenal stress. He routinely measures Secretory IgA from stool samples, and correlates the results with cortisol levels. When there is elevated cortisol there is low or non-existant IgA.

- Raised cortisol is a signal to other cells to go into survival mode, with the result that the body cuts down on enzymes, and digestion is negatively affected. Undigested food attracts fungal activity, and beneficial bacteria are depleted.

- DHEA is another steroid, a sex hormone, which is produced by the adrenals, and converted into testosterone or oestodial. When cortisol goes up DHEA goes down, leading to a maladaptive state. Apart from cutting down on enzymes, the body lays down less calcium in our bones, in order to conserve life-energy.

- Stress also leads to a decrease in mucous secretions, and a reduction in the acidic components of mucous. Bacteria are less able to adhere to the intestinal wall as a result.

- Stress cuts down the movement of food through the digestive tract, encouraging colonisation by more harmful microbial organisms, free to operate when the population of lactobacilli and Bifidobacteria are under threat.

The circular chain of events is hard to break. Add to this the assault of antibiotics, steroids and a high sugar diet, and you have a potent recipe for chronic ill-health. Dr Elias, having seen at first hand the biological effects of stress, insists that you should address the state of the individual, as much as the disease, in order to re-set the body. From his vantage point 'at the coalface' it is easy to see why he is convinced that there is no chronic illness without chronic stress.

Amino acids from protein digestion and the sugars from carbohydrates, plus vitamins and important minerals such as calcium, iron and iodine are absorbed directly into the villi, and then transported to the liver, which acts as a filter. These substances are then released for general circulation.

The colon

The colon or bowel is a long wide tube which starts in the lower right hand corner of the abdomen, then works up and round before coming to an end in the anus. The colon measures $4\frac{1}{2}$ feet, and its function is to move solid material to the anus by peristalsis, or muscle action. It also allows the body to absorb water, electrolytes, and the final products of digestion. But if the walls are blocked by mucous, toxins are absorbed into the body instead. Parasites, yeasts and viruses are encouraged, and the friendly bacteria find it harder to compete. Once the balance is destroyed yeasts and harmful bacteria can migrate to the small intestine and feed on undigested starches and food, causing further fermentation and malabsorption.

Fermentation and malabsorption

When the cells of the body fail to obtain enough nutrients from foods eaten we are said to be in a state of malabsorption. Sometimes excess mucous production, in response to microbial invasion from the colon and their toxins, causes the villi in the small intestine to be 'flattened'. This renders them ineffective in breaking down carbohydrates into simple sugars for absorption. Fermentation is encouraged because of the increased amount of incompletely digested and unabsorbed carbohydrates, providing a food source for candida and bacteria. Moreover, instead of nutrients flowing out into the bloodstream, water carrying nutrients is drawn into the intestinal tract, causing diarrhoea.

By now you may be thoroughly depressed at the seeming impossibility of ever reversing these negative processes. Remember, though, this chapter is merely the beginning of your journey. You will need to learn to nurture and tend your body, rather like a garden. The weeding will involve controlling the harmful bacteria and yeasts. The seeding will involve changing and supplementing your diet, in order to encourage your beneficial bacteria. We will go into more detail about how to do this in later chapters. For now, it is enough to understand why we need these bacteria to ensure lasting health.

Intestinal flora and beneficial bacteria

As we saw in the first chapter, candida is just one part of the body's intestinal flora. These micro-organisms can be divided into viruses, bacteria, fungi and minute single-celled organisms called protozoans. Bacteria and fungi predominate. Our indigenous gut flora consists of 3–4 lbs (1.4–1.8 kg) of bacteria, with 300–500 species, mostly living in the large intestine, or bowel. Our health depends on a delicate balance between these flora.

Probiotics

This term has been adopted to emphasise the positive role that the friendly bacteria play, both nutritionally and therapeutically. One of the most beneficial, yet also most vulnerable, of the bacteria are the *bifidobacteria*. The other major beneficial bacteria are *lactobacillus acidophilus*. Together they are known as the lactic acid bacteria. Their advantages are that they:

- help to maintain the acidic pH in the large intestine, which helps to control pathogens, (disease-causing organisms), including the fungal form of candida.
- deprive other less favourable organisms of oxygen, food and iron.
- enhance the host's digestive and absorptive capacity by helping in the digestion of lactose from milk.
- are thought to lower blood cholesterol.
- regulate immunity.
- are responsible for the synthesis of certain vitamins.
- contribute to more efficient absorption of calcium, phosphorus and magnesium.
- are capable of producing antibiotic products.

Chapter Three

What are the symptoms?

In this chapter we are going to try to make sense of the confusing array of possible symptoms, and how they are produced. The previous chapters provide a basic understanding of what candida is, and how digestion and elimination work. What follows is a more detailed look at what happens to the body when candida gets out of control.

Which symptoms are the most likely to suggest a fungal problem?

One of the difficulties with candida is that the range of symptoms is large, and some could result from causes other than candida overgrowth. However if you have the following symptoms it is likely that candida is a contributing factor to your health problem

- unexplained fatigue
- abdominal bloating and/or flatulence
- food cravings, particularly for sugar and bread
- food and chemical sensitivities
- recurrent thrush and/or cystitis
- rectal itching
- fungal infections of the skin or nails, athlete's foot, psoriasis

Other consequences of candida overgrowth are as follows:

- acne
- endometriosis (disorder of the lining of the uterus)

- headaches
- constipation
- diarrhoea
- abdominal pain
- allergy
- sensitivity to household cleaners, perfumes and tobacco smoke
- recurrent sore throats and blocked nose
- muscle aches
- numbness, tingling and weak muscles
- poor memory, spaced out feelings, irritability, lack of concentration
- premenstrual tension
- ear aches
- joint pain
- blurred vision
- difficulties with weight control – loss or gain
- symptoms worse in damp weather or places
- symptoms worse in mouldy environments
- symptoms worse after eating sugar, yeast or fermented foods
- alcohol intolerance

The brain and candida

When mycotoxins and large food particles are released into the bloodstream, via the leaky gut, they are capable of producing a host of symptoms centred on the central nervous system, such as:

- fatigue
- spaciness
- irritability
- mental fogginess
- memory loss
- depression
- mood swings
- dizziness
- depression

- headaches
- nausea
- burning sensations
- numbness and tingling

Where do symptoms start?

Symptoms usually start in the digestive tract or the vagina, although it is not necessary to have vaginal thrush to have candida overgrowth:

- Bloating and wind are direct results of fermentation in the gut.
- Irritable bowel problems seem to result from food sensitivities, lowered digestive enzymes, sluggish bowel movements, alternating with too rapid transit time.
- Sugar is a laxative, and is an 'expanding' food, attracting water, which does not allow the proper absorption of fluids from the digestive tract to the bloodstream.
- Diets low in roughage also cause problems, because undigested carbohydrates remain in the body longer, and are food source for candida. This increases the fermentation process.
- Food intolerance also causes bowel problems. This leads to mucosal irritation, excess mucous production and disruption of normal digestion and absorption.
- Anal itching is a sign of fungal activity.

Candida in the body

Chronic candida involves the mycelial form of candida and occurs at the stage when the mycotoxins from fungal activity enter the bloodstream.

Chronic candida

One of the problems in accepting the candida diagnosis is the 'implausibility' of attributing so many symptoms to a single cause. Three consequences of faulty digestion and candida overgrowth go some way towards explaining this.

1. Nutrient deprivation. This is caused by malabsorption during digestion, and has long been thought, in other illnesses, to affect the brain causing neurological symptoms. Research on coeliac's disease, caused by an impairment of food absorption from the intestine, is an example here. ('Neurological disorders associated with adult coeliac disease', Cooke, W.T. and W.T. Smith, 1966, *Brain* 89: 683-722.)

   The brain consumes 22 percent of total blood sugar and 25 percent of resting oxygen, making it one of the most nutrient dependent parts of the body. US biochemist, Jeffrey Bland, states that one of the first things that happens in a state of undernutrition is that brain chemistry is affected causing mental confusion, and poor memory.

2. Undigested food particles, and fungal toxins, are given access to the rest of the body via a 'leaky gut'. This is caused in part by the roots of the fungal (mycelial) form of candida which penetrate the lining of the gut whilst foraging for food. This allows undigested food particles and toxins to gain access to the bloodstream, and the liver, which in turn challenges the immune system to go on the alert.

   The food particles are not recognised by the immune system because they are incompletely broken down. They are treated as 'foreign', and as such the immune system tries to neutralise them in order to protect the body. Over time, this situation can undermine immunity, causing allergic reactions, such as asthma and skin reactions, as well affecting the brain.

3. Part of the toxic overload comes from the acetaldehyde effect. This is the chemical that some of us are familiar with when we suffer from 'hangovers'. Candida can produce its own alcohol from fermentation of carbohydrates. Acetaldeyhde, a by-product of alcohol, can overwhelm the liver, and affect the brain.

One of the symptoms of candida is alcohol intolerance. One glass of wine or less is usually enough to tip sufferers over into a drunken state. It is thought that fungi produce a myco-toxin which inactivates the liver enzyme responsible for breaking down alcohol. Trowbridge and Walker (*The Yeast Syndrome*, Bantam, New York, 1987) describe how the acetaldeyde can bind to the cells of the intestine, liver and brain, and liver blood vessels, to their contents such as nutri-ents, enzymes, and vitamins, and to the blood constituents of platelets, leukocytes, erythrocytes and circulating proteins. During extreme acetaldeyde production, these harmful bonds can be formed throughout the body, causing tissue injury.

Chronic candida

The consequences of 'leaky gut' are:

- the absorption of large food molecules into the bloodstream.
- absorption in the same manner of mycotoxins.
- the liver is overworked as a result of toxic overload.
- an immune response, such as asthma or arthritis.
- symptoms of the central nervous system – 'feeling sick all over'.
- general nutrient deficiency.
- chemical sensitivities as the liver becomes overworked.
- lowered defences against viruses and bacteria.
- resulting infections, some of which may linger and can develop into CFS or full-blown ME.
- pain and joint stiffness in varying parts of the body.

It is this final problem which causes confusion amongst health pro-fessionals, because there seems to be no logical explanation for the pattern of change as symptoms shift within the body. However, com-plementary health practitioners suggest that organs which are con-gested have blocked energy, and therefore have diminished immunity. This results from lowered blood flow and reduced oxygen, which may lead to the build up of concentrations of toxic waste resulting in the pain and stiffness. Reducing the candida load can help, as can therapies such as acupuncture, reflexology, shiatsu, reiki and Traditional Chinese Medicine.

Candida and ME

ME (myalgic encephalomyelitis), sometimes referred to as Chronic Fatigue Syndrome, is a chronic disabling disease which affects at least 150,000 people in the UK alone. Although there is usually a viral trigger, with symptoms of chronic infection, some people develop the disease slowly, over time. It is helpful to view a viral 'cause' as a trigger, with many combinations of co-factors which contribute to a process called 'overload'. One co-factor is pre-existing candida problems.

Some candida specialists and practitioners believe that viral activity is enhanced by fungal overgrowth. In one study of 1000 patients with ME 80 percent had had recurrent antibiotic treatment throughout their lives, for ear, nose and throat infections, acne and/or urinary tract infections. There is a great deal of overlap between the symptoms of ME and candida overgrowth, and many people with ME improve on an anti-candida diet, and with anti-fungal treatment.

Candida, food intolerances and food cravings

Those people with food intolerances, as opposed to allergies, have reactions which are slower to take effect, and therefore harder to pinpoint. Many of the symptoms of candida are identical to those found in food intolerance, and are sometimes wrongly diagnosed as a result. Thus one of the major symptoms of intolerance to food or inhaled substances is fatigue. However, concentration solely on food intolerance as cause, without investigating gut permeability, can be short-sighted.

Testing for food intolerance if you have a candida problem is something to consider, and it is certainly important to reduce intolerance as part of the treatment. As treatment progresses however and the gut wall heals, food intolerance should reduce although there may be *some* foods which you should avoid or rotate indefinitely. Often these foods are dairy products, gluten, tea and coffee.

In a recent study in the *Lancet* gluten, found in wheat, rye, barley and oats, was not tolerated in three-fifths of the 53 patients with Chronic Fatigue Syndrome who were tested. Some of the symptoms were alleviated when they cut out these foods from their diet. Gluten sensitivity causes inflammation of the small bowel lining and neurological symptoms due to degeneration of the peripheral nerves and the spinal chord.

Food cravings often accompany food allergy or intolerance. This is because our bodies tend to crave the very foods which are causing the most problems. Thus many candida sufferers crave sugar and bread. Once these foods are cut out of the diet, after some initial withdrawal symptoms, the 'need' for those foods dies down. The body is then better able to free itself from mood swings which fluctuate from high to low, and the accompanying fatigue.

Hormonal interactions and candida symptoms

Hormones are chemical messengers which travel via the bloodstream. They regulate automatic responses, bring together bodily functions and form part of the endocrine system.

There is a connection in the body between the immune system, the nervous system and the endocrine system. Underlying many candida problems may be adrenal insufficiency. Our adrenals become exhausted following: bacterial or viral infection; mental and emotional stress; poorly regulated blood sugar levels; and/or a state of dietary deficiency. Adrenal problems can lead to a weakened digestive system; allergic responses to food; an increase in general sensitivities; decreased body metabolism; increased muscle breakdown and an increase in fat deposition.

More women than men are vulnerable to candida problems; indeed, naturopath Leon Chaitow and one of the first authors to write about candida in the UK, describes women as the main candida targets (*Candida Albicans: Could Yeast Be Your Problem?*, Thorsons 1996.).This is thought to be due to the hormonal fluctuations that women experience every month (and the over-use of antibiotics for vaginal and bladder infections as well as use of the pill and HRT.) Certainly, more women have candida problems between puberty and the menopause than before or after.

Candida has an affinity to both oestrogen and progesterone, two female hormones. The higher blood sugar levels associated with higher levels of progesterone in the second half of the menstrual cycle could be the reason for a corresponding increase in candida symptoms around that time. (See Dr Luc de Schepper's book *Candida, The Symptoms, The Causes, The Cure*, Foulsham, 1990.)

Candida albicans can produce an adrenalin-like substance that can affect heart muscle, leading to a rapid pulse. Research also shows that low blood pressure is commonly found in those with candida problems. Blood pressure can be normalised by the use of anti-fungal drugs, thus demonstrating a possible connection.

Auto-immunity

Auto-immunity is the process whereby the body's own immune system attacks parts of itself, causing a reaction. Auto-immune diseases such as rheumatoid arthritis, lupus and multiple sclerosis are examples of illnesses which sometimes respond well to an anti-candida diet and programme.

Minerals and candida

Anaemia is sometimes a consequence of candida overgrowth. This is because candida can compete for limited supplies of dietary iron.

Zinc and magnesium deficiencies are also commonly found. Zinc is needed to defend against viral activity. Magnesium plays an important role in energy production and muscle function.

Bacterial and fungal interactions

Toxic shock syndrome can be fatal and is caused by the bacteria *staph aureus*. However, experiments have shown that this bacteria is not fatal on its own, but that when combined with candida albicans it becomes virulent, and far more potent. Some researchers are convinced that mixed bacterial and fungal co-infections are the most advanced and severe stage of infection, and consequently the most difficult to treat.

Candida and mercury amalgam

The main source of mercury in the gut is from amalgam fillings. Recent research shows that mercury vapour disturbs the balance of the gut flora, and certain gut bacteria, including candida, become progressively more resistant to mercury, and to eradication. This is based on laboratory tests which show that if you find an appropriate antibiotic for an appropriate organism and then repeat the test, but add mercury to it, then the antibiotic no longer achieves its effect. Composite or 'white' fillings can be used to replace mercury amalgam, but they are more expensive.

Which comes first?

Does candida cause problems with immunity and other bodily systems, or do problems with immunity lead to candida overgrowth? The answer is probably both. Whichever way round is correct, a holistic approach, involving nutrition, diet, anti-fungal supplements, exercise, together with spiritual and emotional therapies, seems, on the basis of sufferers' experiences to help reverse problems of yeast overgrowth. The next chapter gives guidelines on testing and diagnosis.

Chapter Four

Testing and diagnosis

This chapter looks at methods of diagnosis for candida-related problems. This is not easy, because until recently there was no one test which could be relied upon. This is because stool tests used to assess the size of candida colonies do not always give an accurate picture. Various others are listed below. The lack of a reliable test has not helped increase the acceptability of candida overgrowth as a diagnosis with doctors.

As a result, many practitioners prefer to rely on noting the patient's symptoms and careful history taking. The diagnosis is either confirmed or denied by their response to treatment, which is usually a change of diet, combined with anti-fungals and probiotics. Those with candida overgrowth usually start to feel better on a change of diet, but the introduction of the anti-fungals is likely to cause symptoms to increase in the short-term because of the effect of 'die-off'. This is the effect on the body of toxins released from dead candida cells.

It is also possible to build up a reasonable picture of what is going on by obtaining tests for different aspects of candida overgrowth, such as:

- stool test
- saliva test for female hormone levels and imbalances
- adrenal stress index
- gut permeability tests
- glucose tolerance tests
- alcohol fermentation tests
- food intolerance tests

- tests for hydrochloric acid levels in the stomach
- acid/alkaline tests
- hypothyroid test (low thyroid test)

Most of these tests are only obtainable through a practitioner and few are available on the National Health. However, the hypothyroid test can be done at home very easily:

The hypothyroid test

Take and record your temperature for 10 minutes before you get out of bed in the morning. You should do this for a minimum of three days, including, if you are a woman, days 2 and 3 of your period, although for greater accuracy you should continue over the whole of your monthly cycle. If the temperature is below normal then hypothyroidism is likely, and should be checked by a doctor. Low thyroid function causes fatigue, weight gain and thinning of hair. There is a connection with this problem and stress, because cortisol controls thyroid production.

Complementary health tests

There are further tests not usually acceptable to scientific medicine, but which nevertheless, in experienced hands, are of considerable use. Most have evolved from 'energy medicine' – where the body is seen as a series of interacting energy fields, which can be used to diagnose, with a variety of different 'routes' to access what is going wrong. Some of them are:

- Traditional Chinese Medicine such as acupuncture – which uses deep pulses and the condition of the tongue.
- Electro-dermal techniques – such as the Vega machine.
- Iridology – which diagnoses illness by 'reading' the iris of the eyes.
- Reflexology – which believes that every part of the body is linked to points or zones on the feet by meridians (energy lines).

- Kinesiology: Touch For Health – which uses muscle testing to detect energy blockages, and meridian energy flow.
- Healers – who use their hands to detect changes in energy fields.

Some of these diagnoses and examinations may use terms which do not refer directly to 'candida overgrowth', but do give indications of imbalances and related consequences. Thus Chinese medicine refers to 'heat' and 'damp' inside the body, and 'stagnant energy'. Candida is a damp condition which needs more digestive 'fire'. This makes sense when we think of fermentation and mould (damp), coupled with digestion which is sluggish and inefficient (cold, without energetic impulse). Looked at in this perspective, candida is not seen necessarily as a cause, but as a symptom of other underlying problems to do with energy flow, best addressed with a total programme of holistic care, involving diet, herbs, working directly on the body with needles or pressure, exercise, and meditation.

In iridology it is possible to 'see' in the map of the iris, excess mucous production in the intestines. This would add to other indications of fungal overgrowth, from symptoms. If necessary, a further test for gut permeability could be done, or a stool test for candida and parasites.

Candida Questionnaire

If you suspect you have a candida problem it is best to start by answering a questionnaire, which gives the main symptoms. The following questionnaire was devised by Dr Crook and adapted by Jane McWhirter for continuing use as treatment progresses. She added two columns for ticking off symptoms during and towards the end of treatment. We suggest you fill in this questionnaire and refer back to it as you get better. Once they begin to get better, most people forget how bad they felt when they were ill, before changing their diet, and taking control. It's a boost to recognise how far you have come, even if you still have some way to go.

Dr Crook's Candida Questionnaire

Underline the questions below that apply to you and add up the score at the end of section A. Make sure you have dated it as you will want to refer back in 6 weeks and 6 months time and re-score to check on progress.

Section A: History   Date _____

Point score

1 Have you taken tetracyclines or other antibiotics for acne for one month or longer?   35

2 Have you, at any time in your life, taken other broad spectrum antibiotics, for respiratory, urinary or other infections for two months or longer, or in shorter courses four or more times in a one-year period?   35

3 Have you taken a broad-spectrum antibiotic drug - even a single course?   6

4 Have you, at any time in your life, been bothered by persistent prostatitis, vaginitis (thrush) or other problems affecting your reproductive organs?   25

5 Have you been pregnant:
2 or more times?   5
Once?   3

6 Have you taken birth control pills:
For more than 2 years?   15
For 6 months to 2 years?   8
Have you been on an IVF programme?   25

7 Have you taken prednisone or other cortisone-type drugs:
For more than 2 weeks?   15
For 2 weeks or less?   6

8 Does exposure to perfumes, insecticides, (dry cleaners or petrol stations) or other chemicals provoke:
Moderate to severe symptoms?   20
Mild symptoms?   5

9 Are your symptoms worse on damp, muggy days or in mouldy places?   20

10 Have you had athletes' foot, ringworm or other chronic fungus infections of the skin or nails? Have such infections been:
Severe or persistent?   20
Mild or sporadic?   10

11 Do you crave sugar?	10
12 Do you crave bread?	10
13 Do you crave alcoholic beverages?	10
14 Does tobacco smoke really bother you?	10

Total score section A ....

Section B: Major symptoms

For each of your symptoms, enter the appropriate figure in the point score column:

If a symptom is occasional or mild:	3 points
If a symptom is frequent and/or moderately severe:	6 points
If a symptom is constant and/or disabling:	9 points

Add the total score and record it at the end of this section.

	Now	In 6 weeks	In 6 months
1 Fatigue (unexplained) or lethargy			
2 Feeling of being drained			
3 Poor memory			
4 Feeling spaced out or unreal			
5 Inability to make decisions			
6 Numbness, burning or tingling			
7 Insomnia			
8 Muscle aches (or tenderness)			
9 Muscle weakness or paralysis (or cramps)			
10 Pain and/or swelling in joints (Stiffness in the mornings)			
11 Abdominal pain			
12 Constipation			
13 Diahorrea			
14 Bloating, belching or intestinal gas (wind)			
15 Troublesome vaginal burning, itching or discharge (thrush)			
16 Prostatitis			
17 Impotence			

	Now	In 6 weeks	In 6 months
18 Loss of sexual desire or feeling			
19 Endometriosis or infertility			
20 Cramps and/or other menstrual irregularities			
21 Pre-menstrual tension			
22 Attacks of anxiety (panic, depression) or crying			
23 Cold hands or feet and/or chilliness			
24 Shaking or irritable when hungry			

Total score section B ....

Section C: Other symptoms

	Now	In 6 weeks	In 6 months
1 Drowsiness			
2 Irritability or feeling jittery			
3 Lack of co-ordination			
4 Inability to concentrate			
5 Frequent mood swings			
6 Headaches			
7 Dizziness/ loss of balance			
8 Pressure above ears/ feeling of head swelling			
9 Tendency to bruise easily (or heal slowly)			
10 Chronic rashes or itching (or acne)			
11 Numbness, tingling			
12 Indigestion or heartburn			
13 Food sensitivity or intolerance			
14 Mucous in stools			
15 Rectal itching			
16 Dry mouth or throat			
17 Rash or blisters in mouth			
18 Bad breath (or foul taste)			
19 Foot, hair or body odour not relieved by washing			

	Now	In 6 weeks	In 6 months
20 Nasal congestion or nasal drip			
21 Nasal itching			
22 Sore throats			
23 Laryngitis, loss of voice			
24 Cough or recurrent bronchitis			
25 Pain or tightness in chest			
26 Wheezing or shortness of breath			
27 Urinary urgency or frequency			
28 Burning feeling on urination (cystitis)			
29 Spots in front of the eyes, or erratic vision			
30 Burning in the eyes, or tears			
31 Recurrent infections or fluid in ears			
32 Ear pain or deafness			

Total score section C ....

Total score section A ....

Total score section B ....

GRAND TOTAL SCORE ....

Scores will vary depending on whether you are a man or a woman:

Women	Men	Yeast-connected problems are:
180	140	almost certain
120	90	probable
60	40	possible

Chart © William Crook. Reproduced from
The Practical Guide to Candida (McWhirter, 1995)

Taking control, and finding help

Bear in mind that the questionnaire is a starting point for professional diagnosis and is *not* an invitation to self-treat. You should consult your doctor to rule out other causes. You may be reluctant to do this if you have already done so, and failed to get appropriate help. However, if you did not connect your various symptoms together, you may not have mentioned them all.

Even if your doctor is sympathetic and willing to listen to your self-diagnosis, you will not necessarily get the help that you need. Some will prescribe antifungal drugs, others may suggest antidepressants, but very few have the time, or the training, to help you combine candida control with the necessary dietary approach to healing and long-term recovery. Most of the doctors who treat candida are in private practice, and have come to specialise in nutrition after their traditional medical training. This means that if you have a candida-related problem, you are likely to have to pay for treatment.

Therapies, outside the traditional medical field, which are particularly helpful in treating candida overgrowth are naturopathy, herbalism, and nutrition. These are base-line therapies, upon which you can add other therapies as you get better. They all share a holistic perspective which means that they take account of the body-mind-spirit connection, and the effects of the environment on health.

Because of the large amount of work that you will be required to put into getting better you will need to see your relationship with your practitioner as a partnership. Guidance and help from outside is essential, but in the end *you* are doing to have make the changes, and take stock of your lifestyle.

Chapter Five

Treatment: restoring the balance

Throughout this chapter bear in mind that how quickly you respond to the treatment programme, and the pace at which you follow it, will depend on the level of your problem with candida. If you have chronic candida with wide-ranging toxicity, you may need careful monitoring, a rigid approach to the diet, and an intensive supplement programme. If you have only recently become ill, candida will be less invasive, and the underlying imbalances in digestion and absorption easier to clear up.

Old ideas and new beginnings

But first, some misunderstandings which need to be addressed, for those who followed an anti-candida programme before some of the newer supplements and treatment programmes were devised. Unfortunately, many of these people have begun to doubt the 'candida' hypothesis for two reasons:

- Although they got better when they followed a strict diet, they failed to come off this maintenance regime without getting ill again. It became a diet for life.
- After taking antifungal drugs for many years some found they were worse when they came off the drugs than they were before. Anti-fungal drugs, such as nystatin, only kill a small number of candida strains, leaving others resistant, and hardier than before. When the drugs are stopped, the prob-

lems re-surface in a more chronic form. Certain parasites may also have gone untreated.

We have had to refine our understanding of what is going on, and to tailor treatment to not only 'destroy the bad guys' with the newer and more effective natural anti-fungals, but also to heal the gut wall, and re-seed with beneficial bacteria. This deeper and more fundamental approach to treatment takes account of our immunity and how to foster the ecology of the gut. These strategies work long-term alongside basic changes in eating habits and life-style.

Changing your environment

- You may find you react to perfume sprays or common household cleaners which contain chemicals – experiment by cutting down on chemicals in the home, and buy non-perfumed products.
- Static electricity from nylon carpets is sometimes a problem. Consider natural alternatives.
- Check out your tolerance of house dust. Do you need to change your bedding to hypo-allergenic pillows and duvets?
- Household plants sometimes harbour mould. You may feel better if they are loaned to a friend for a while. If your symptoms are worse in the autumn because of leaf mould you may need to protect yourself from over-exposure. Deal with mould problems in the house, under sinks, and so on, especially if your symptoms are worse in damp weather.

Finding a practitioner

Once you are ready to find someone to help you, join a support group to talk to others further along the path to recovery than you, to find out what the practitioners in your area have to offer. Jane McWhirter's book, *The Practical Guide to Candida* (1995) includes a directory of practitioners listing qualifications, experience, fees, and a brief description of what they do. Some parts of the country have fewer resoures than others, but that does not mean that there is no-one in your area. Ask in local health food shops, or write a letter to your local newspaper, asking for other sufferers to contact you. Phone up and talk to your chosen practitioner yourself, explaining what you think your problems are, in order to get a feel of whether you can work in partnership together. Is this practitioner going to give you enough time? Can you contact him/her by phone if you have severe 'die-off' or toxic reactions? Can they give you the emotional support you need, or would you need to look elsewhere?

Practitioners generally fall into two groups when it comes to treating candida. There are those who are firm about the 'rules' of treatment, and who manage to get compliance by telling you what to do, and giving a long list of supplements. They may not have so much time for listening, or for taking account of your anxieties. The second group depend as much on the quality of the therapeutic relationship, as strict adherence to a set formula. Encouraging you to to take responsibility and to get to know your responses when you do eat the wrong foods is part of the treatment, rather than simply insisting that you stick to the rules without question. You need to decide what kind of practitioner suits your personality and your needs.

The candida programme

This programme outlines how candida overgrowth and gut dysbiosis are treated, in partnership with a skilled practitioner.

Whilst we list here the nutritional requirements of many with candida problems you need to recognise individual variations, and levels of absorption. If you have a mild candida problem you may find some of the supplements listed here unneccessary, because the core part of the candida programme, a change of diet, with antifungals and probiotics, is enough. On the other hand, for those who have been ill for some time, and are stuck, having tried the above, there may be something in this list which could make all the difference.

Previous medications

If you are on any prescribed medication, do not stop taking it without first consulting your GP. (For a discussion about natural alternatives to over-the-counter drugs read Jane McWhirter's *Practical Guide to Candida*. It is full of useful information and advice.)

Food intolerances

If candida overgrowth has been diagnosed by a practitioner, and other conditions have been excluded by your doctor, the next step is to test for food intolerances. Your practitioner will give you guidance on this. However, it is likely that the anti-candida programme will lessen food sensitivities over time.

Support for the pancreas and the liver

It is also helpful to ask for an assessment of organ weakness, using muscle testing, the Vega machine, or other diagnostic tools. This is important because of the likelihood of liver and pancreatic stress over the period you have been ill. Herbs to support the liver are silymarin (milk thistle), dandelion, artichoke, turmeric, ginger root, goldenseal. HEP 194, a herbal combination product from BioCare, is particularly effective. If taken at this stage the body will be better able to tolerate candida toxins once you start to take anti-fungals. For the pancreas you can supplement with pancreatic digestive enzymes. Those of vegetable origin are best. They are particularly helpful for bloating, diarrhoea, or constipation.

Detoxification

Some candida experts recommend a detoxification fast at the start of the programme. However, it may be more sensible to follow a more gentle regime, unless you are closely observed by your practitioner.

Dry skin brushing

Start the day by helping your lymph system's ability to detoxify. Do this by dry skin brushing before you bath or shower. You can buy a brush for this purpose from health food shops, chemists or mail order companies. Start with the legs and feet, using gentle circular actions at the groin, and long, firm strokes towards the heart. Move on to your arms and hands, particularly the lymph nodes under the breast muscles. Cover the rest of the body where possible, and finish with the stomach, moving up on the right and down on the left. Now you are ready for an invigorating shower.

Probiotics

At the same time as starting the main candida control diet, it is important to start taking probiotics. Probiotics are concentrated sources of beneficial bacteria, and as such are a way of replacing the indigenous benefical bacteria of the gut which will have been depleted if you have candida problems. Unfortunately the benefical bacteria found in live yoghurt are not numerous enough to make much difference. The best probiotics contain lactobacillus acidophilus and bifidobacteria, because they are normally resident in the gut, and will adhere to the gut wall if it is not inflamed. The best products should have instructions to refrigerate, and should be encapsulated to protect from damage from moisture in the air. BioAcidophilus, from BioCare, is acid-stable, which means that it survives the acid environment of the stomach before implanting lower down in the digestive tract. It is compatible with human strain bacteria, unlike some probiotics which use beneficial bacteria derived from animal sources. Each capsule contains 4 billion microbes.

Gwynne Davies, a leading candida practitioner (naturopath and kinesiologist), and candida workshop lecturer, has found that starting his patients off with BioCare's Replete (20 billion microbes per day) for one or two weeks, has cut treatment time down from six or nine months, to three months. After one week of Replete, follow up with BioAcidophilus. However, the manufacturing process for Replete is complex, and the product is costly; nearly £30 for a week's supply, at current cost. If your budget is tight, and your condition is mild, cut out the Replete, and just take an ordinary probiotic, which is half the price. Combine with Enteroplex, (a combination of cabbage extract (Vitamin U) and licorice) if your gut wall is sore and inflamed. This will help the probiotics to adhere. Although you may find the smell from the concentrated cabbage extract unpleasant, it is worth persevering.

Anti-fungals

After six weeks on probiotics, introduce anti-fungals, whilst carrying on with the HEP 194 to support the liver. You may need to lower the dose if the 'die-off' is severe, building up gradually until you can tolerate it once more. ('Die-off' refers to an increase in symptoms from the release of toxins from the dead candida cells, caused by the anti-fungal treatment.)

Natural anti-fungals

Garlic
Garlic concentrate, or fresh raw garlic, is a natural antifungal, which is also antibacterial and antiviral. It acts systemically, which is why you notice the smell on your body if you have eaten a large amount.

Put one chopped or minced (not pressed or crushed) clove of garlic on the back of the tongue, and wash it down with water, without chewing. Do this during a meal, rather than on an empty stomach. Dr Zoltan Rona, a medical doctor, and co-author of an American candida diet book, reports that she has excellent results this way, but do not continue for longer than three months at a time to avoid sensitivity developing. Remember to use organic garlic.

If you prefer your garlic in supplement form choose a product which retains the natural Allicin content through freeze drying. Blackmore's Garlix is effective.

Candicidin
Candicidin was the first non-chemical anti-fungal to be manufactured which is effective systemically beyond the digestive tract. Others are broken down as food substances before they have a chance to act beyond the gut wall. Candicidin is comprised of plant oils from oregano, cloves, artemisia, ginger and borage seed, in a base of grapefruit seed oil and lauric acid. Extensive trials have confirmed that it is effective against E. coli, salmonella, all strains of candida, Capylo bacter and H. pylori.

Caprylic acid
Caprylic acid is a short-chain fatty acid found in human breast milk and coconuts. This is an effective anti-fungal, but it is important to find one which is time-released, so that it reaches lower down into the large intestine. Mycopryl, in different strengths, is time-released. Some people, especially those with ME, find its action quite strong, and they may need to try something more gentle.

Berberine
Products containing Berberis and Golden Seal are an ideal alternative for those who cannot tolerate Mycopryl, because they contain berberine, which normalises the natural bacterial content of the gut, at the same time helping the immune system.

Combinations
Another successful antifungal which is gentle in its action is CG233, or Colon Guard. It combines garlic, caprylic acid, butyric acid, lauric acid, aloe vera and biotin. Biotin helps to control yeast cell division. Although this product was devised as a maintenance product for use after treatment, some practitioners are having excellent results at the beginning of treatment when it is combined with Eradicidin Forte.

Eradicidin Forte
If your liver finds it hard to cope with 'die off' (toxins from reducing candida overgrowth) you could leave probiotics until a later stage, and use a herbal combination product, such as Eradicidin Forte. It contains Artemisia Annua, Berberis and grapefruit seed extract. It has antiviral, antifungal, antiparasitic and antibacterial properties, and is gentler in its action than other more specific antifungals.

Olive oil
Cold-pressed virgin olive oil contains a substance called oleic acid, which has antifungal, antiviral and antiparasitic properties. Because it is absorbed in the small intestine its activity overall is restricted. Nevertheless, taking six teaspoons a day with food is recommended.

Grapefruit seed extract
Grapefruit seeds have antiparasitic and antifungal properties. Different formulations come in different strengths, and in capsule or liquid form. Even if you are intolerant of citrus foods, you would be able to tolerate the seed extract. This is best combined with garlic supplements.

Rotation
If you are environmentally sensitive, or highly allergic, you may need to rotate antifungals over a four or seven day period, with different combinations each day.

Anti-fungal drugs

Some doctors prefer to use anti-fungal drugs, such as nystatin (Nystan) and flucanazole (Diflucan). In fact, it is not necessary to use them without first trying the new and effective natural anti-fungals.

There is a danger, particularly with nystatin, that long-term use merely destroys a limited number of strains of candida, allowing other resistant strains to remain unchecked. If you are given anti-fungal drugs, make sure that equal attention is paid to repopulation with beneficial bacteria and healing the gut wall. If you find it hard to come off nystatin, you could be helped by combining it with a natural anti-fungal.

Healing the Gut Wall

There is no point in taking probiotics if at the same time you do not pay attention to your gut wall, which, if the candida has changed into its fungal form, will be damaged by penetrating hyphae or roots. Practitioners will differ on the stage at which these supplements are introduced as supplements. Choose from:

- Butyric Acid, a short-chain fatty acid found in butter and olive oil which helps maintain the natural barrier.
- Combinations which include N-Acetyl-glucosamine (NAG), an amino sugar which helps in reconstructing tissue damage, and which assists friendly bacteria to adhere to the gut wall.
- L-glutamine, an amino acid which supports gastro-intestinal growth.
- Gamma-oryzanol, or rice bran oil, which is soothing for gastrointestinal inflammatory conditions
- Fructooligosacharides (FOS) – sugars that occur naturally in vegetables and other plants. They are beneficial because they encourage healing of the gut wall, and recolonisation of Bifidobacteria.
- Enteroguard, a combination product, with added zinc, magnesium ascorbate, and Vitamin A.

Essential Fatty Acids (EFAs)

Essential Fatty Acid supplements, such as Mega GLA work as anti-inflammatories, and help maintain the integrity of the cell wall. (See page 79 for further explanation of EFAs.)

Nutritional supplements for strengthening immunity

Nutrients which are particularly beneficial within the candida programme for building immunity are: vitamin C, vitamin E, vitamin A, selenium, zinc, iron, copper, folic acid, vitamin B12, vitamin B6, magnesium, and calcium.

If you tolerate nutrient supplements poorly in the early stages of treatment, gradually build them up until you are used to them. Gillian Hamer is a nutritionist, practitioner and lecturer based at all Hallows House in the city of London. She has a down-to-earth, common sense approach, coupled with sound grounding in science. She prefers to use a single good multivitamin and mineral supplement, feeling that this is better than trying to compensate for deficiencies with individual supplements. For non-pregnant women she suggests a special formula called FemForte from BioCare. In addition she prescribes GLA Complex for its anti-inflammatory effects.

Antioxidants

Oxidation is a loss of electrons, when there is not enough free hydrogen. It leads to the ageing process and is the cause of reduced immune function and disease. Antioxidant enzymes, hormones and nutrients have the job of neutralising free radical damage and could be a key factor in recovery, especially if your yeast problems persist and lead on to chronic fatigue. Antioxidants also help with food sensitivity. You need to use a broad range of antioxidants for them to be effective. (For a factsheet on Antioxidants write to Action for ME enclosing stamps to the value of £1 and a SAE) Microhydrin (the Wellbeing Company) is particularly effective, and is the only antioxidant which does not itself become a free radical. It also helps with acid/alkaline balance. See Candida Workshops website for further information.

Chromium

If you have low blood sugar you may benefit from supplementing with Chromium.

Parasites

Treating for candida seems to reactivate formerly dormant parasitic infestations. With candida overgrowth there is usually a corresponding low stomach acid problem, which encourages parasites. There is now a reliable stool test for parasites. If, as is likely, you develop this problem towards the end of treatment, try the Chinese herb, Artemisia. The combination product Artemisia Complex is a good source, because it also includes echinacea, for immunity, and licorice for healing the gastrointestinal tract.

Digestive aids

Candida treatment will cause added stress to digestion, and you will probably require digestive aids. One holistic doctor with a busy practice treating candida found that 75 per cent of her patients, on testing, had low stomach acidity. Betaine and pepsin hydrochloride, and glutamic acid hydrochloride all helped. There is no toxicity or dependence involved, and the stomach eventually learns to increase acid production on its own, once exposed to these supplements.

Treating vaginal thrush

During the cleansing process initiated by the *Beat Candida Diet*, and anti-candida supplements, many women may find that their vaginal thrush gets worse. Dead yeast organisms, especially those colonised around the sexual organs, are eliminated through vagina, causing vaginal discharge. It also seems that the vagina is the one of the last areas to respond to diet, needing local treatment as well. It is important to know how to manage this problem by creating an acidic environment for the friendly bacteria to take hold. A vagina which is too alkaline could encourage candida to recolonise.

- Douche with a weak solution of apple cider vinegar, with one part vinegar to three parts distilled or purified warm water, to acidify the vagina. Jane McWhirter recommends adding to the solution three drops of Tea Tree Oil, three drops of Lavender Oil, and three drops of Rosemary Oil. To obtain a douche you can ask a chemist for a plastic syringe or use a meat baster. If you still have a problem obtaining a douche, you can soak a small natural sponge in the solution and leave in the vagina for several hours or overnight, or lie in a bath with cider vinegar added.

- Try douching at different times with Oxy-Pro (BioCare), a potassium/sodium compound that releases oxygen at the site of application. Use 10 drops diluted in just under a litre of purified water. Yeasts do not thrive in well oxygenated cells, and this has a direct effect on any organisms that may have colonised the area. Douching allows whatever is used to penetrate higher than creams or pessaries. Liquid grapefruit seed extract is an effective alternative to use as a douche.

- Cervagyn cream (BioCare) can provide relief from minor vaginal irritations. It contains 3 per cent potassium sorbate, combined with olive oil and camomile. This helps the symptoms of swelling, itching and discharge.

- After a week or so of acidifying the vagina with the apple cider vinegar, insert two acidophilus capsules in the vagina each night. Prick each capsule several times with a pin just before inserting to release their contents once in place. Do this for one or two weeks.

- To prevent infection and reinfection from a partner, use a condom.

- For men who have penile thrush, try a cream called Dermasorb, which combines acidophilus with Tea Tree Oil.

Reinfection from the throat

When anti-candida treatment stops, some people find that their symptoms return because their gastro-intestinal tract is being re-seeded with candida from the throat. Gargle with Oxy-Pro, a potassium/sodium compound that releases oxygen at the site of application. Swallow for additional benefit against candida in the upper intestine.

Taking time to switch off

Calming the mind, through relaxation and meditation, is a real benefit in the healing process. Try to create the right environment – give yourself time to feel comfortable and free from distractions of people, noise and telephones. There are many useful relaxation tapes on the market to guide you through the various stages.

Meditation

Meditation is a way of resting the mind. It helps, however, to be taught how to do it. (See page 213 for details of clinically standarized meditation tapes) Reaching a point where you can see yourself healthy and happy during meditation is a sign of progress.

Autogenics

Autogenics is a practical form of stress management which is accessible through training in individual or group sessions. Once taught, the exercises are easy to do anywhere and anytime. It involves directing your attention inwards and focusing your mind on phrases relating to different parts of the body, in the following way:

- sensations of heaviness in your body
- warmth in your arms and legs

- your calm and regular heartbeat
- your easy and natural breathing
- warmth in your abdomen
- coolness in your head.

Changes of circulation and temperature occur in the areas of the body focussed on. It also helps with pain control, relaxation and better sleep.

T'ai Chi Ch'uan

T'ai chi ch'uan has often been called 'meditation in motion'. It is thought to have been developed out of a blend of Taoist philosophy and the martial arts in eleventh century China. It involves learning a series of slow movements to encourage energy flow, and toning and massage of internal organs.

Yoga

Yoga is suitable for all ages and levels of fitness, and is one of the most complete mind-body therapies there is. You will be taught the correct way to breath, and given gentle stretching movements and postures which will gradually extend your suppleness and energy levels. Like t'ai chi, yoga will also help your mental state, with profound psychological benefits.

Maintenance after recovery

Gillian Hamer encourages her clients to continue taking a multivitamin and multimineral combination, together with GLA Complex and vitamin C. For the first month she will suggest CG233. Every three months, in addition, she recommends a course of probiotics, such as BioAcidophilus. These measures should ensure that candida problems are kept under control.

You are probably thinking that all this is enough, more than enough, to get to grips with. But underpinning everything that you do, think and feel is how and what you eat. The next section deals with the diet connection, and how to make the changes that will lead to sustained and lasting recovery.

Summary of the candida control programme

- Herbal support for the liver.
- Plant based digestive enzymes
- Detoxification with gentle fasting, followed by the *Beat Candida Diet* for six weeks, or move straight to the diet.
- Take a broad-based yeast-free multi vitamin and mineral supplement. FemForte (BioCare) is especially good for women.
- Extra Vitamin C is a good idea.
- Take GLA Complex every day (Essential Fatty Acids).
- Lemon water on waking.
- Dry skin brushing.
- Whole linseeds for colon health.
- Start taking probiotics once following the *Beat Candida Diet*.
- After six weeks on the *Beat Candida Diet* start antifungals.
- Include products to heal the gut wall - follow guidance from your practitioner regarding when to introduce these.
- Treat for parasites towards the end of the programme, if appropriate, with Eradicidin Forte.
- Maintenance: carry on with a multivitamin and mineral, GLA Complex, and Vitamin C, and introduce CG233 for the first month. Take probiotics every three months.

Part II

The Healing Power of Food

Chapter Six

The principles behind the *Beat Candida Diet*

Whilst those who are sick often need to come to terms with changing their eating habits, doctors are still geared to the concept of clinical disease arising from some individual genetic susceptibility, or outside pathogen. They have so far been slow to acknowledge that many of the major public health disorders affecting us today have a dietary connection. When the public are encouraged to think of improving diet, the focus is usually on the problems associated with the excess intake of saturated fats and trans-fatty-acids. In fact, there is a general nutritional deficiency in the population as a whole which is a direct result of imbalance in our diets, and the adulteration of food from chemicals and pesticides.

The answer lies in the soil

At the turn of the century very few doctors thought that health and disease were related to diet. Disease was understood instead to originate from micro-organisms or toxins. Future treatment would preferably involve antitoxins, chemicals or vaccines. The disease/diet connection, so neatly illustrated by the reversal of scurvy with Vitamin C from lemon juice, was forgotten in this frenzy of scientific excess.

But during the same period, Dr Robert McCarrison was studying the people living in the Hunza valley in the Himalayas looking for explanation of their extraordinary long lives, free from disease, and their perfect physique. Their healthy diet of grains, vegetables and fruits, with milk and butter, and goat's meat on feast days, was an important factor, but he discovered that what made them different to other groups of people was their use of manure, made from organic waste – human and animal excreta, vegetable scraps, and ashes from their fires – and combined with soil made rich with glacial silt.

As Barbara Griggs points out in her fascinating book *The Food Factor*, this immunity from disease was found in later experiments to be passed on to cattle fed on disease-free crops. The crops had been grown following the principles of eastern methods of cultivation with organic waste. Insects and fungi, already shown to be resisted by crops, were unable to take hold on cattle fed with such grains.

There are two lessons for us in this. There is not just a con-nection between health and the kind of food we eat. *How* the food is grown is also vital. What the food is able to take up from the soil gives protection from disease and determines what that food in turn is able to give back to our bodies.

Thus the first principle in the *Beat Candida Diet* has to be the importance of organic food. Chemical fertilisers, insecticides and fungicides rob food of essential trace elements, which in turn rob us of what we need to stay healthy and thrive. If you are trying to return your body to a state of healthy equilibrium, then you have even more need for the curative power of health-giving, live organic food.

BUT (gut) reaction:
'*But* organic food is more expensive.'
'*But* where can I buy organic food?'

'*But* I haven't got time to go out of my way.'

'*But* vegetables from the supermarket look better and last longer.'

Food fact: In tests done in 1991 organophosphate residues were found in carrots. The Ministry of Agriculture, Fisheries and Food (MAFF) now advises consumers to peel non-organic carrots to avoid the danger of consuming pesticides. Eighty-five per cent of the food value of carrots is in the skin.

Beat Candida Diet reaction:

- If you are cutting out processed and ready-made foods for the *Beat Candida Diet*, does it cost more to substitute organic food? The diet cuts down on the amount of animal protein at each meal, so that buying organic meat and wild fish should not cost more, given the proportion that they will form overall in each meal, with vegetables. At least, make a resolution to eat only organic carrots, onions and potatoes. These are available in many supermarkets.

- Investigate box schemes in your area, where you have delivered to your home a weekly box of seasonal pre-selected organic vegetables. More and more health-food shops are meeting the competition by providing this service as well. Stock up your freezer with organic meat.

- You save time with a box scheme. It can be satisfying and worth the extra time involved to go yourself to buy from an organic farm. Knowing how and where your food is produced gives an extra dimension to healing foods. Can you really justify eating mange-touts from Kenya, knowing that the pesticide levels are so high that farm workers are being permanently damaged?

- An increasing number of supermarkets include a range of organic foods. Make sure the store manager knows of your interest. The more consumers speak up about what they want the greater the demand will be for produce. The greater the demand, the greater the likelihood that eventually the prices will decrease.

- Try the blindfold taste test with an organic and a non-organic carrot. Invest in a bristle vegetable scrubbing brush. That natural coating of soil will help to remind you that food comes from the earth rather than a factory with artificial and standardised outcomes.

Food fact: The 'cheap', chemically, mass produced, and intensively farmed food that we are dependent on bears a hidden cost, not just to the environment, but also to the consumer. Salmonella poisoning costs the national purse £23.4 million each year, based on 1988–89 figures. BSE (bovine spongiform encephalomyelitis) cost £700 million, with a further £3.3 billion set aside to protect public safety and restore consumer confidence in beef. Joanna Blythman in her book *The Foods We Eat* (Michael Joseph, 1996), calls this 'nothing less than a quantifiable economic and social catastrophe caused by the brinkmanship of industrial farming.'

The yin and yang of food

In Chinese philosophy the terms 'yin' and 'yang' have been used for thousands of years to describe how the world works. Yin and Yang, whilst being part of a whole, are also opposites, pulling in different directions. A good example of this is the definition for male and female characteristics. They are only understood when looked at in relation to each other, and an acknowledgement is made that each contains elements of the other. Combining these two extremes leads to balance and wholeness.

In relation to food, yin and yang would be translated as expansive (yin) and contractive (yang). Both are needed by our bodies, and being aware of this provides a useful compass when cooking. Animal products, such as beef, pork, lamb, poultry, eggs and fish, and salty foods, are contracting. You may notice that when you eat them you feel more tight and closed. On the other hand foods with sugar in them, such as fruits, most dairy products, cakes, sweets etc are expanding foods.

Think back to when you ate too much salt. Salt is contracting to the body, because it draws water to it. Did you then crave
something liquid and sweet, such as orange juice, which is
expansive, to correct the balance? Women before their periods
are often 'contracting' and become constipated as a result. Sugar
cravings at this time are common, in an attempt to 'open' or
relax enough to shed the lining of the uterus, and in response to
an increase in progesterone levels which encourages yeast overgrowth. You may at this point be lulled into thinking that if
sugar is 'relaxing' it could be a good thing! Finding a way,
through diet, to bring your body back into balance, without the
ups and downs, (and resulting candida overgrowth) that come
with sugar, is a better alternative. As you will see, it is possible to
create food choices which correct the contraction and expan-
sion tug-of-war.

When we crave 'expanding' foods we are trying to get back
into balance, but really we are setting in motion a see-saw which
undermines our health. We need to encourage foods which are
neither one nor the other, but are naturally balanced – plenty of
salads and vegetables. Contracting foods are fine, as long as their
total quantity is reduced, and balanced with the natural sweetness from onions, carrots and squashes. See Donna Gates' book
The Body Ecology Diet for a further explanation of this principle
in relation to candida.

BUT (gut) reaction

'This sounds fine in theory, *but* in the meantime how do I deal
with my sugar cravings? Or other cravings, for that matter?'

Beat Candida Diet reaction

- To help with sugar (and bread) cravings put 1 tablespoon (15
  ml) of apple cider vinegar or lemon juice into a glass of warm
  water and drink twice a day.
- Eat little and often, with snacks between meals, to regulate
  blood sugar levels.
- Supplement with Chromium
- Try the amino-acid L-glutamine, separately from food.

> *Acid-forming foods*
> Animal proteins (such as meat, cheese, fish, eggs), grains (except millet), bread, sugars, pasteurised milk
>
> *Alkali-forming foods*
> All vegetables (potatoes, if cooked in their skins, and if the skins are eaten), sea vegetables, salads, fresh fruit (except plums and cranberries), almonds and unpasteurised milk.

Acid/alkaline balance

We have already talked about the importance of acid/alkaline balance in Chapter 2. Many people with problems of yeast overgrowth have a condition which is too acidic; yeasts, viruses, and other parasites thrive in an acidic environment. The underlying cause of most disease is the wrong chemical condition in the body which the body cannot eliminate. When the results of digestion and metabolism are too acidic, problems start to happen. Constipation is the main cause of acid formation.

To maintain the acid/alkali balance there should be approximately four times as much alkali-forming food as acid-forming food. This is a ratio of 80 percent alkaline-forming food to only 20 per cent acid-forming food. To attain this you should increase the quantity of vegetables you eat. (Fruits, despite their alkaline-forming value, are generally restricted, or eliminated, on anti-candida diets.) You need to reduce acid-forming animal proteins, starchy foods and nuts (except almonds). Sugar is already eliminated for other reasons. Millet is the only grain

Practical tip
To aid digestion and to avoid the temptation to overeat or eat too fast, place the protein content of the meal in a small bowl, with vegetables heaped on the plate. Take small amounts from the bowl (Chinese-style) as you progress through the meal.

which is not acid-forming. Not surprisingly, this perspective dove-tails neatly with the expansion/contraction theory. By reducing animal products (contracting and acidic) in this way, you are doing yourself a favour all round.

Food combining

How different foods are combined at the same meal is an essential component of the *Beat Candida Diet*, because food combining leads to more efficient digestion. As we have seen throughout this book, if you can improve your digestive processes you inhibit candida overgrowth, and encourage beneficial bacteria. Although this may seem to add further complication to an already overcrowded programme, you do not have to see this as something to practice permanently. You can try it for three months, have a break, and then come back to it when you feel you need to.

This system of eating goes against everything that many consider 'normal'. Out go cheese sandwiches (which are not part of the *Beat Candida Diet* anyway), out goes meat with potatoes, out go fish and chips, out goes pizza. These combinations are considered inappropriate because they mix in the same meal concentrated proteins and concentrated carbohydrates. Meat can be eaten with neutral foods such as non-starchy vegetables and salads. Potatoes are eaten separately from meat, and also with vegetables and salads.

Food Combining was first developed and written about as a way of eating for health by Dr William Howard Hay in 1935. He believed that toxicity and acid waste products that built up in the body could lead to disease. He recommended that proteins be cut down, along with starches and heavily processed foods, and that vegetable and fruit consumption should be increased. He also saw that separating foods that do not digest well together allows the body to use the food we eat more efficiently. In subsequent years Doris Grant has written widely on this way of eating, her *Food Combining For Health*, written with

Jean Joice is a classic, and recently the books of Kathryn Marsden have made Food Combining even more accessible. (*The Food Combining Diet*, Thorsons, 1993)

This way of eating draws attention to the fact that proteins and carbohydrates require different acid/alkaline mediums for digestion. Proteins are the largest molecules in the body, and need to be broken down into amino acids in an acid medium in the stomach. Carbohydrates are broken down into sugars in an alkaline medium. If carbohydrates are mixed with proteins, the stomach acid is partially neutralised, causing the proteins to be incompletely digested. This then provides food for fungi and other bacteria. Where there is a mixture of both types of food neither food is properly digested, which may lead to fermentation.

Protein foods are all kinds of meat, all kinds of fish, soya products, dairy products (cheese, milk, yoghurt), nuts, seeds and eggs.

Starchy carbohydrates include grains (wheat, oats, rye, rice, barley, buckwheat, millet), pasta, flours, and products made from these, and some starchy vegetables, such as potatoes. Complex carbohydrates refer to the wholegrain variety. Refined carbohydrates, such as white sugar and flour, and potatoes without their skins, do not contain the nutrients needed to aid digestion, and rob the body of other nutrients.

Neutral foods are vegetable and salad foods which mix with either proteins or starches. Thus meats can be eaten with vegetables and salads (neutral), and vegetables and salads can also be eaten with starchy carbohydrates, like grains, pulses or potatoes.

Fruit should be eaten alone, away from proteins or starches, or before a meal, so as not to hinder digestion. This is because fruit requires a much shorter time to digest, and this could hasten the digestion of protein if eaten together, leading to incomplete digestion and fermentation. However fruit is limited on the *Beat Candida Diet*, although it can be gradually increased towards the recovery phase.

Keeping proteins and carbohydrates separate also helps to regulate the acid/alkaline balance. This is because, according to Dr Nadia Coates, fewer starchy foods are required by the body because those that are eaten are used more efficiently.

Pulses, such as dried beans, chickpeas, and lentils, contain both protein and starch, and present a problem for the food combining rules. However, if prepared properly, with adequate soaking, and renewal of the water for cooking, they do provide a valuable source of protein for vegetarians, and meat eaters who need a wider variety of protein. For food combining purposes they are best eaten on their own or with salad or vegetables. If you sprout pulses, they become mostly predigested proteins. You will need to sprout for at least two days. See Leslie Kenton's book *Raw Energy* for more information on sprouting. The best pulses are mung, lentils, aduki beans, flageolets and chickpeas.

Water Another aspect of food combining, and the *Beat Candida Diet*, is adequate water intake, apart from meals. It should be filtered, or bottled, and at room temperature. It helps, after the dehydration of sleep, to take at least half your daily intake of fluids by mid-morning.

Cleansing and detoxification

Following the guidelines in this book to control candida, and normalise digestion, takes time, effort and patience. You should also be prepared for the consequences of your actions; the release of accumulated toxins in your body may result in you feeling unwell, or the temporary increase in some of your symptoms. These toxins will not just be those released by the dead candida cells, but also waste and poisons stored in body tissues over the years.

It is important that your organs of elimination are given extra nutritional support, especially during the first three months when reactions will be strongest. The main organs of elimination are the lungs, the liver, the kidney, the skin and the colon. Herbs for the liver are very important. A 'healing crisis' often occurs when toxins are released from fungal colonies and dumped into the system, having been stored in body tissue over time. This happens naturally as the body starts to heal itself. You may start to get headaches, loss of appetite, nausea, fevers, fatigue, skin eruptions and swelling of lymph glands. When toxins are released into the bloodstream, they need to be removed by bile from the liver. If the intestines are sluggish the toxins will be reabsorbed, causing overload in the liver.

To prepare you for this difficult time, we suggest that you ease yourself into the *Beat Candida Diet* by following Stage 1: The 2 Week Action Plan beforehand. You may repeat this for a longer period of time if you wish. This will give you a chance to lessen the strain on your detoxification pathways, and give you time to get used to the new foods, and new ways of eating. When you are ready to follow the stricter anti-candida diet, with antifungals, your liver will be be better able to cope.

Here are some tips for helping detoxification and cleansing in Stage 1:

- Take cold-pressed olive oil to stimulate the gallbladder – neat or in salad dressings.
- Skin brush.
- Increase your intake of raw garlic.
- Soak 1 tablespoon of organic linseeds in water overnight, and swallow before breakfast, with plenty of water, for added roughage and to avoid constipation.
- Try colonic irrigation, but only with a qualified therapist.
- Give yourself plenty of relaxation and rest.
- Make a point of getting outside for some of the day in natural light and fresh air.

The next chapter goes into detail about which foods will help on the *Beat Candida Diet*.

Chapter Seven

Star foods for recovery

Making the right food choices is the best way to start the process of healing for gut dysbiosis and candida overgrowth. Even when you introduce antifungals and supplements to heal the gut wall, diet is a cornerstone of management, and should not take second place to nutritional supplements.

In this chapter we intend to give you an understanding of which foods are helpful on the *Beat Candida Diet*. We have called the foods that positively work against candida 'star foods'.

Finding a balance between eating as 'medicine' and eating for pleasure or convenience if you have been used to eating in ways which have contributed to your ill health, is not easy. You may take a while to get used to some of the foods which we highlight. Many recoil at the thought of sea vegetables (seaweed), despite the fact that they have been a significant component of traditional diets quite near to home, (Ireland and Wales) as well as abroad, particularly in Asia. In the recipes we give you the option of using strong flavours or unusual ingredients in ways which do not overpower other tastes, but which do contribute nutritional benefit. But you do have a choice. For example, garlic may not be your favourite food. In that case, leave it out of the recipes, and take garlic capsules, or rely on other antifungal supplements instead.

The message that we want to get across is that this section of the book is not written in stone. You can play around with the recipes, taking out foods which do not agree with you, and substitute with those that do. We provide the guidelines here, and within these there are various levels for you to stick to, depending on the severity of your health problems and your particular personality.

As far as the *pace* of change is concerned, we recommend that you give yourself plenty of time to move into the diet, and the treatment. (If you cannot tolerate some of the warming foods we highlight – spices such as cayenne and ginger – move forward in other directions and come back to them later in small doses, allowing time between each experiment.) Taking your time fits in with the pace best suited to your body. Your body needs time to adjust, and you need time to reorganise your life so that you are meeting your needs with gradual commitment, once you have worked out how to put everything into place. Rushing into this programme is a recipe for disaster, unless you have large reserves of energy and outside support. Ask yourself whether your personality dictates that you have to do something 'perfectly' from the word go. Does that lead to automatic success, or does it mean that sometimes you give up when things start to go wrong?

The *Beat Candida Diet* is not an invitation to martyrdom. Feelings of deprivation have no value here. The aim is to move to a place where eventually what we need to eat matches what we freely choose and enjoy eating. The flexibility within the guidelines is for you to experiment with, and also acknowledges that we are not superhuman. 'Breaking the rules' does not mean that you return to the starting post. It is this coming back and forth which will eventually allow you to appreciate how your food preferences have changed. And how, as your body gets into balance, you are stronger and more able to tolerate a wider range of foods.

Star foods

Garlic

Hippocrates, the father of modern medicine, recommended the use of garlic for infectious diseases and intestinal disorders.

The medical properties are contained in the garlic oil, or allicin, which is also responsible for the anti-social smell of garlic when crushed. Apart from antifungal, anti-candida yeast properties when eaten raw, garlic increases absorption of vitamins, and thins the blood. It is also a decongestant, and therefore excellent at dispelling mucous.

Garlic produces a marked effect on the intestine, helping diarrhoea, and colitis, and aiding in the elimination of toxins. It stimulates peristaltic action, and the secretion of digestive juices, and kills harmful bacteria, whilst not affecting the beneficial bacteria.

Food fact: Chewing fresh parsley seems to purify the breath after eating raw garlic.

Cook's note: You can roast or boil the whole clove, unpeeled and uncut, then squeeze out the garlic pulp and add to the recipe. Or, cut off a thin slice from the pointed top end of the bulb and the aroma will automatically pass to the other ingredients. Garlic cooked whole has a rounder flavour which is more acceptable to some palettes. The more you use the rounder it gets. Although in cooking you rob the garlic of most of its beneficial effect, we also recommend garlic for the flavour it gives to food!

Onions

Onions are one of the oldest cultivated vegetables. Raw onions are more easy to digest than fried or cooked onion. However, for natural sweetness to balance other tastes in a meal, you should fry onions slowly for some time. Blanching onions is a good idea. Onions are rich in calcium and riboflavin. They help water retention and mucous build-up, and are beneficial for the heart.

Daikon

Daikon is a long white radish, sold in many greengrocers and supermarkets, and used by Chinese cooks. It helps to maintain a healthy balance of beneficial bacteria, and is good for the digestion of oily foods. It can be grated as a side salad with a few drops of wheat-free tamari on its own, or with grated carrot. Keith Michell in his book *Practically Macrobiotic* advises not to throw away the daikon greens – they can be steamed as a green vegetable.

Fish

Fish is the best source of animal protein if you are not vegetarian. Fish found in natural cold, deep-water habitats provide the most nutritious essential fatty acids. Wild (not farmed) salmon, trout, fresh tuna, fresh sardines, mackerel, eel and cod are rich in omega-3 fatty acids, which are an essential component of the *Beat Candida Diet*.

Food fact: Farmed salmon is very cheap and tempting to buy. Unfortunately, you get what you pay for. Restricting fish to cages causes flabby, drier fish, and a uniform diet which takes no account of species' preferences breeds flavourless flesh. Because living in close proximity increases the likelihood of disease, farmed fish are continually exposed to antibiotics. They are also fed artificial pink colouring to enhance the colour of their flesh.

Cook's note: Fish is as versatile as chicken but for best results cook it quickly. Cooking methods which the *Beat Candida Diet* recommends are steaming, baking in a parcel, grilling or stir-frying. Baking preserves the essential fatty acids more effectively than grilling or frying.

Lemons and limes

The lemon is a valuable antibacterial food, which plays a prime role in the list of healing foods. It is useful for killing fungi in the mouth and throat, although its antifungal effects are limited further down the digestive tract because by then it gets broken down and absorbed. There is a common misconception that lemons are acidic. In fact they are alkaline. The lemon has a higher level of vitamin C than the lime. Both are too sour to feed the candida, and are therefore an acceptable fruit. Whereas oranges (which are acid-forming) often cause problems of food sensitivity, lemons and limes are usually well tolerated by most people with candida problems.

The juice of both lemons and limes make a good tasting combination with garlic, ginger and olive oil – many dressings and marinades in the *Beat Candida Diet* are based on this winning combination.

Food facts: Lemons and limes are waxed to prevent deterioration in storage. If you use the zest of waxed fruit, scrub the rind well under running water before grating. Organic lemons are not waxed. If you are sensitive to lemons substitute cider vinegar for lemon juice where appropriate.

Essential fatty acids

Fatty acids are the basic building blocks of fats and oils. Three of these fatty acids – *linoleic acid, linolenic acid* and *arachidonic acid* – are polyunsaturates. They are essential for growth, and regulate many body processes. They are called *essential fatty acids* (EFAs). A diet rich in EFAs ensures healthy cell membranes, thus giving protection from viruses, bacteria and fungi. One of their functions is also to conduct electrons and energy through the cell molecule. Linoleic acid is an omega 6 fatty acid and Linolenic acid is an omega 3 fatty acid.

Linolenic acid and arachidonic acid can be obtained from food, but are also synthesised from linoleic acid. Linoleic acid is only obtained from the food we eat, and is therefore a vital component of our diet. It is easy to become deficient if we are not careful. Linoleic acid deficiency has been linked to eczema and psoriasis, hair loss, infertility, growth deficiency, weight disorders, immune deficiency and circulatory disorders.

Linoleic acid can be found in safflower oil, brown rice, sweet-corn, avocados, pumpkin seeds, sunflower seeds, sesame seeds and sesame oil. The necessary step, in the body, to convert linoleic acid to gammalinoleic acid (GLA) needs zinc, magnesium, vitamin B6 and biotin. These are nutrients which are usually in short supply for those with candida problems.

Trans-fatty-acids are harmful impostors, almost unknown in nature, which have been introduced to the body by modern food processing techniques associated with fats and oils. They block the action of EFAs, weakening the cell membrane, and admitting substances such as allergens, undigested foods, viruses, fungi and potential carcinogens. They also inhibit the production of GLA. It therefore makes little sense to consume vast quantities of trans-fatty-acids, from stabilised and adulterated oils and hydrogenated margarines (Vitaquell is one good alternative).

GLA is one of the nutritional requirements we strongly recommend candida sufferers to supplement with. The source that most of us have heard about is evening primrose oil. A more concentrated source, is to be found in GLA Complex, from BioCare (19.5 per cent as opposed to 9 per cent). The highest concentrated source of all is in mother's breast milk (22.4 per cent). GLA Complex also contains squaline, an oil that helps stimulate the immune system.

Olive oil

Olive oil contains oleic acid, a monounsaturate, which is valuable in the control of candida, because it prevents the transformation of candida to its mycelial form. It is the best oil to use as a dressing on salads and foods. That is, as long as it is traditionally pressed, and sold in opaque containers or tins. If the bottle is transparent, store it in the fridge in anything that will block the light. When cold it may go cloudy, but once back to room temperature the cloudiness will disperse.

Of all the oils, olive oil is subjected to the mildest form of processing, but because of that it is more vulnerable to degredation, according to Dr Robert Erdmann, author of *Fats, Nutrition and Health*. This is because polyunsaturated acids are very sensitive to heat. So when it comes to cooking, you should choose between more stable oils, with short chain saturated fatty acids, such as butyric acid (butter) or palmitic acid (coconut oil). They are more stable, and do not react adversely with air and heat. Butyric acid is a valuable source of healing for the gut wall. Try not to worry about the fact that these fats are saturated. Indians have been using ghee (made from butter) for centuries. (And the Chinese way of stir-frying, traditionally, was too minimise oxidation with polyunsaturated oils by putting food and oil together before heating.) If you wish, you can increase the stability of olive oil for cooking by adding ghee. (See below.)

'Extra virgin' denotes the first pressing of the best quality olives, without processing, so it has the highest oleic content and fullest flavour of all the olive oils. It retains its vitamin and mineral co-factors. 'Virgin' implies the first pressing of good but not best quality olives, without processing. As the pressing continues, processing, called refining, will be introduced to remove the bitter tang the stressed fruit releases. Oil labelled 'pure' means a mix of first and second pressing. 'Cold pressed' denotes that no heat has been used in the pressing process, although the pressures and frictions involved in pressing are enough to heat the oils. 'Extra virgin' is the best choice to make for flavour, health and the scent of olives, although you will not be getting an oil that lasts very long. The cheapest oils are fully refined, de-natured, nutritionally empty, chemicalised, deodorised, and everlasting (not life-giving) oils. They are odourless and tasteless. The price you pay will be your health and your recovery.

Ghee

Ghee is clarified butter, which is simply what is left from butter once the milk solids have been removed. It can be combined with olive or coconut oils for frying and sauteing. Concentrated butter sold in supermarkets has added milk powder, but ghee sold in tins in Indian- and West Indian-run shops, or supermarkets, is fine.

Linseed oil (flaxseed oil)

This is the best source of the Omega 3 essential fatty acid, linolenic acid. Previously in the UK its healing properties were used only on cricket bats and horses, but it is now produced to food quality standard, although finding the required standard, from a health point of view, is not easy. It should be sold in an opaque bottle, and stored in a cool, dark place to be eaten within three weeks. It can be added cold to hot food once cooked, or used instead of olive oil for salads or mayonnaise. It is also available emulsified in stabilised capsules.

If you cannot obtain a good quality oil, use organically grown seeds instead. You will need three times the quantity of seeds to oil. We have already described the use of soaked seeds as an aid for regular bowel movements. To benefit from the soaked seeds, chew them so that digestive juices can release the essential fatty acids. You can also process them, for example, in a coffee grinder. Use them freshly ground, rather than storing extra seeds for future use. They can also be added to cereals, and other food.

Almonds

Almonds, known as the king of nuts, are a highly nutritious food, containing high levels of almost all the trace elements needed by the body. They are an excellent source, like olive oil, of oleic acid, linolenic acid (100 grams of almonds contains 11 grams of linolenic acid), of vitamin E, and boron (effective against bone density loss in osteoporosis). They are a good alternative plant protein, particularly when pre-soaked or sprouted. Almonds, unlike other nuts, are alkaline, and when soaked and sprouted combine with any foods. To sprout, cover the whole nuts with bottled water in a jam jar with a muslin cover held in place with a rubber band. Leave for twelve hours. Drain for 8 hours. Store in the fridge, and consume within two days. See our recipe for almond milk, an excellent substitute for cow's milk, although be aware of the high fat content of almonds. Do not overuse them.

Seeds – sunflower, sesame, pumkin

These seeds are a good source of protein, vitamin E, B (except B12), fibre and unsaturated fats. Although seeds are easier to digest raw than roasted, you could try dry roasting them (in a frying pan without oil, stirred frequently), and adding to salads. Sunflower seeds can be given extra flavour by stirring in some wheatfree tamari after roasting. Sunflower seeds can also be soaked and sprouted in the same way as almonds to add to cereals, salads, or as a nutritious snack. Try sprinkling over vegetables to augment their protein, vitamin and mineral content.

Some candida sufferers are said to have a problem with sesame seeds. Always buy from a reliable source, to ensure freshness.

Ginger

Ginger has long been renowned as a 'medicine of the stomach', and is effective against nausea and sea-sickness. Ancient physicians used ginger as a carminative and anti-fermenting medicine. Its heat is good for reducing mucous, chesty coughs and all cold and flu symptoms.

It is preferable to use the fresh ginger root, than ginger in powder form. Peel the knobbly root, and either slice it thinly and fine chop, or grate on the coarse side of the cheese grater. Japanese shops, and some health food shops, sell purpose made ceramic ginger graters, with an indentation to extract the grated ginger juice by pressing.

Make yourself some fresh ginger tea at any time you need a lift, and appreciate its warming and soothing properties. Grate and squeeze ginger juice into a saucepan with water. Boil gently for ten to twenty minutes.

Herbs

Herbs that are particularly healing are cayenne, coriander, cumin, turmeric, ginger and garlic. Cayenne stimulates the secretion of hydrochloric acid. Cumin has warming properties, and is good for digestion and wind. Turmeric, contains curcumin, which is an anti-inflammatory agent and antioxidant.

Cider vinegar

Raw, unfiltered cider vinegar is recommended on the *Beat Candida Diet*, although most other fermented foods are not. It should be sold in dark, light-proof bottles. It is rich in potassium, and is antiseptic and alkaline forming, which means that it provides the right environment for beneficial bacteria. Some people may find that it irritates their digestive tract; they should give it a rest for a while and return to it later. An alternative is to take it with oil in a dressing, where the effect is buffered, and less able to cause problems.

Cooked or raw? Hot or cold?

- Although raw foods contain more enzymes and vitamins, and are beneficial, many people with candida problems cannot digest them easily. If this is your problem, rely more on soups, and lightly steamed or stir-fried vegetables.
- Raw cider vinegar, and unsalted, raw, cultured vegetables (as in naturally fermented sauerkraut) provide plant enzymes, which may be lacking if you cannot tolerate raw food.
- There is no great value in cooked food from the point of view of absorbing amino acids, enzymes and vitamins. Digestion time will more than double to 7–10 hours with the loss of enzymes. Putrefaction, and colonisation by fungi is likely to follow. The *Beat Candida Diet* encourages you therefore to begin the process of digestion of meat and fish by using a marinade. A simple mixture of lemon juice, crushed garlic and olive oil poured over the meat some 20 minutes to 8 hours in advance of cooking will break down the connective tissue. This applies

particularly to all darker meats. This 'soaking' will also enhance the flavour and succulence of the foods which will aid digestion.

- The value of cooked food, apart from being palatable and comforting, is that minerals are released, and fibre broken down. Vegetables which are slowly steamed or stir-fried release their minerals quickly.
- Starting a meal with something hot will slow down digestion. Therefore, start some meals, if you can tolerate it, with something raw (eg. grated carrot, or daikon with olive oil and garlic). This will generate the production of hydrochloric acid and the digestive enzymes needed to breakdown the more complex cooked food to follow.
- Eating seasonally, and in tune with the weather, is a good idea. Increase warming cooked foods in the winter, and in the summer, as you get stronger, eat more raw vegetables and salads.

Sea vegetables

Otherwise known as seaweed, these foods are full of iodine, which governs the thyroid gland. They also contain an acid which prevents pollutants from being absorbed by the body. Another advantage is their fibrous quality, which cleanses the colon, and their ability to promote acid/alkaline balance. If you are worried about cutting out dairy products, and losing out on calcium, use sea vegetables to compensate. At the same time you will be building up your sources of zinc.

To start with, try nori flakes for sprinkling on food, or Japanese sushi with sheets of nori. Add Kombu strips when cooking pulses to make them more digestible. Apart from the recipes here, you will find many more which use sea vegetables in macrobiotic cookbooks. Your health food store will be another source of information. You can balance their salty taste by cooking sea vegetables with sweet vegetables, such as onions and carrots.

Vegetables

'Vegetables in the Middle East do not play second fiddle as do the "two veg" to meat in England. They hold a dignified, sometimes splendid position in the hierarchy of food. They are, in turn, mezze, pickles and salads. They can be stuffed and ranked as a main dish, an adornment to meat in a stew, or deep fried, sauteed, or steamed. In cooking, their nature is taken into account, and their flavour, texture and colour are treated with respect. They are expected to give of their best.' *Book of Middle Eastern Food*, (1968) Claudia Roden.

In Britain we are burdened with the view that vegetables are 'good for you' rather than pleasurable. We are also unimaginative as to how to combine vegetables with herbs and spices to make them even more interesting. Now that you are going to increase your vegetable consumption, it is even more important that you prepare them in ways which are appetising and delicious. Starchy vegetables should not be overused, and some candida books are cautious about beetroot, despite its beneficial use for the liver, because of its high sugar content.

Broccoli, Brussels sprouts, cauliflower and cabbage

These vegetables are all members of the *cruciferous* family, and contain high levels of vitamin C, beta carotene, folate, iron and potassium. Include these vegetables in your diet daily if possible. By cooking them in the minimum of water, steaming or stir-frying some of the high vitamin C content will be retained. Use the cooking water for soups and sauces. Best of all nibble raw and serve in summer salads.

Cook's note: Stocks from cooked vegetables should be stored in the fridge for no longer than 48 hours. After that bacteria will turn the water cloudy and foul smelling. Instead, freeze some once cooled, for later use.

Chapter Eight

Foods to avoid, foods to choose

Before we look more at the wider range of foods available on the *Beat Candida Diet*, we need briefly to consider those foods that *do not* help with combatting candida overgrowth. This may be the most depressing part of the book for some. However, we finish this chapter with plenty of alternatives and suggestions, in order to end on a positive note. Whilst you will need to cut out sugar for the longest time, perhaps indefinitely, you may be able to reintroduce yeast products after three months, as you get better. Gluten, primarily in wheat, is seen increasingly to be a major problem in candida overgrowth. You should seriously consider cutting out wheat to evaluate your response. It may be possible to tolerate it on a rotational basis later.

Foods to avoid

Sugar

All carbohydrates eventually end up as glucose and other simple sugars circulating in the bloodstream. Complex carbohydrates take some time before they are degraded into glucose, whereas simple carbohydrates and sugars are broken down very quickly. This latter process leads to large fluctuations in the levels of blood sugar in the blood stream, and resultant insulin surges to control them.

Apart from the strain this puts on the pancreas, other problems follow: endocrine problems, hormone imbalances and altered body chemistry, all induced by sugar consumption. This is reason enough to cut down sugar, but sugar is cut out on the anti-candida programme because it encourages yeast overgrowth. Sugar and refined carbohydrates are foods for yeasts. They also provide you with no nutritional benefit to justify their use.

Avoid all sugar, and foods which contain them, to include:
- honey
- molasses
- maple syrup
- sugar substitutes
- quick acting carbohydrates such as sweets, cakes, biscuits
- alcoholic drinks
- milk sugar (lactose) from milk products
- some tinned food
- fruit sugar from melons and grapes, and other high sugar fruits
- fruit juices – although freshly pressed apples can be added to home-juiced vegetable juices in small quantities, as a substitute for carrots.

Food fact: Butter contains only small amounts of lactose, and is therefore allowable, in small quantities. Live yoghurt left to ferment for long enough has very little lactose left, and is encouraged on the *Beat Candida Diet* because of its beneficial effect on the environment needed for lactic acid bacteria. However, these live bacteria in yoghurt do not implant. You still need to supplement with probiotics. Because of widespread intolerance to dairy foods, you may find goat's and sheep's milk is better. It is also less intensively farmed than cow's milk, and should contain less drug residues

Fruit: the grey area

Practitioners have varying attitudes to fruit and candida. Some ban it entirely, except for lemons and cranberries. Others suggest you have no fruit for the first three weeks, and then gradually introduce it, on its own, limiting it to two pieces a day. Gillian Hamer takes the 'relaxed' approach, which can be tightened up according to response. She recommends a broader range of choices: bananas, apples, pears, mango, pawpaw, and avocados, as well as lemons for dressings and in drinks. Oranges are not part of the *Beat Candida Diet*. They are highly allergenic for many people.

Food fact: Lemons and limes, unlike other fruits, can be eaten with other foods such as salads, fish and other animal protein. Some people however find the combination of lemons and grains hard to digest.

Yeast

Candida overgrowth seems to cause an allergic reaction to yeast, often suggested by symptoms such as bloating and wind. For the first three months avoid all yeast-based foods, after which test your reaction upon reintroduction. Eliminate yeast for one week and then eat it two times in the same day. Leon Chaitow recommends that you check for reactions such as fatigue, brain fog, palpitations, or other symptoms which were previously absent. If you have no reactions, introduce yeast on a rotation basis of once in four or five days only for three months.

Foods which contain yeast are as follows:
- breads
- cakes
- yeast spreads, such as Marmite
- biscuits and crackers
- pastries, buns, rolls
- stuffing mixes, and products with breadcrumbs (fish fingers, etc)
- mushrooms
- soya sauce (wheatfree tamari is naturally fermented and OK)
- all cheeses, particularly hard cheeses (with the exception of soft vegetarian goat's cheese).
- all dried fruits
- all fermented drinks, such as beer, spirits, wine, cider
- all malted products

- foods containing monosodium glutamate
- vinegars
- miso, tempeh, tofu
- smoked meats and fish, processed meats – contain yeasts
- nuts not in their shells, or not freshly opened. Avoid peanuts altogether.
- foods which are not fresh (be careful about storage time in the fridge)
- nutritional supplements which are not labelled as yeastfree

Food fact: Two exceptions to the above limitations are organic raw, unfiltered apple cider vinegar, and raw, unsalted sauerkraut, both alkaline-forming, and beneficial for the ecology of the gut. If you find you are sensitive to these foods, cut them out and try later. Try combining the apple cider vinegar with olive oil.

Food fact: Modern baker's yeast has been genetically engineered to by-pass the slower, acidic bacterial stage of fermentation. Natural 'wild' yeasts, used in sourdough breads, or naturally leavened breads, are acid tolerant and therefore co-exist happily with beneficial lactic acid bacteria resident in our digestive tracts.

Gluten

Gluten is found in wheat, and to a lesser extent in rye, oats and barley, but not in millet, rice or most types of corn. It seems that problems for health have arisen mostly from the alteration to the chromosome structure of wheat to make it more suitable for the intensive cultivation methods of modern agriculture.

In wheat the nutrients used to be in the wheat germ, but in modern wheats, over the last sixty years, the nutrients are in the outer part. Because the ear is exposed, with no beard coverage, the most important part of the grain is unable to defend itself against fungal contamination. Another difference is that before the bran was soluble, but now it is toughened and unbreakable, rather like PVC. Storage of grains also causes problems. This is because of the problem of drying vast quantities sufficiently well to avoid fungal contamination.

Gluten is a sticky viscous protein which causes problems when transported into the blood, through a damaged gut wall. It is not a true recognisable protein, and as such can be seen as an allergen by the body. This is because the modern varieties of wheat do not break down in the same way as wheat varieties before hybridisation. Having gained access to other bodily organs, such as the liver, spleen, pancreas or gall bladder, gluten causes disturbances in function. It sticks to anything, and in this way transports into the blood insufficiently digested sugars, cholesterol, fats or salts.

It is easy to see, therefore, that wholewheat is not so much of 'a good thing' as we are led to believe because of the toxicity of the bran, and the high levels of proteins and hormones of fungal origin. In those with an allergic response a large number of white blood cells are produced. Together with gluten, they lead to excess mucous production, a trap for undigested food, and a food source for fungal, bacterial and viral organisms growing in the gut. A recent study in the *Lancet* has confirmed the potential of gluten to cause problems in the body. Research shows that gluten can interfere with neurological pathways and cause illnesses of the brain, such as schizophrenia.

Gluten intolerance

Gluten intolerance affects digestion, causing abdominal rumblings, water retention, weight gain, fatigue, and gritty eyes. The possibility of a 'yeast connection' to gluten intolerance is strong, and confirmed by most practitioners working in this area, and many who came to our workshops. Dr Nadia Coates, a pioneer in alerting others to the dangers of gluten intolerance, suggests that it may follow milk intolerance in childhood.

Again, there are differences of opinion when it comes to diet as to whether all gluten should be cut out, or just the high gluten grains such as wheat. We suggest the latter option. Certainly, it is worth trying to include oats in your diet. It does not contain gliaden in its gluten content, and this may be why it is better tolerated. It is important to keep your options open for a wide dietary choice, but at the same time be alert to food reactions and tolerances.

Hydrogenated margarines

Hydrogenation is a process used to solidify vegetable oils in the manufacture of margarines, which damages fatty acids, and undermines health. One brand of margarine which does not use the hydrogenation method isVitaquell. It is usually available in health food shops.

Refined carbohydrates

You will need to avoid all refined carbohydrates, such as white flour, white rice, refined pasta. This is because their sugars are too fast-acting, causing insulin peaks and troughs, and sugar cravings. Refined food does not carry within it the nutrients for its own digestion, and therefore robs the body of nutrition which it may not have in reserve.

All stimulants and nicotine

Tobacco is heavily processed and contaminated with fungal residues. Inhaling nicotine robs the body of oxygen which should be available to body cells. People with prematurely lined and wrinkled faces are usually smokers.

Coffee and tea, even decaffeinated, are not part of the anti-candida programme because of their addictive qualities and their affect on the adrenals. It is better to cut these drinks out entirely whilst you are trying to overcome candida. Your immune system needs sustainable energy, not artificially boosted by the short-lived highs from caffeine. The high tannin levels in tea can also cause iron depletion if drunk to excess.

Foods to choose

You will see from the recipes we have selected that there is a wide range of foods to choose from. Indeed, the recipes cannot possibly cover every option. We have already highlighted those foods which are especially beneficial for healing your gut wall, and controlling candida. We list here some others which are permissible. Some may not agree with you for individual reasons. You may need to experiment, or get help from your practitioner to eliminate poorly tolerated foods. Often they can be reintroduced later.

Yeastfree breads

Naturally leavened sour dough bread, such as the Russian Rye bread, is available in many supermarkets, or via mail-order. Sprouted sour dough rye, which is lighter, will provide extra roughage because the whole grain is used. This is a moist loaf, and very good toasted. You can also make your own soda bread using Spelt flour. Although this is wheat it is from an ancient variety, without some of the problems engineered into modern varieties.

Meat and poultry

It is best to buy organic meat because of residues of antibiotics and hormones present in intensively-farmed animals. Of the non-organic meats, lamb and wild game are the safest. Chicken is a highly contaminated meat, owing to the way it is mass pro-duced. If you cannot afford to buy organic chicken because of the quantities you consume, substitute with non-animal protein, and buy chicken less often, or use smaller quantities which can be cut up for stir-fries.

Potatoes and other starchy vegetables

Opinions differ about the value of potatoes. Some feel that their high starch content encourages fermentation. Our view is that they are a useful food, but caution needs to be used and you should not eat them every day. Experiment with grains in order to rotate and diversify. Parsnips are also very starchy. We have used them in the *Beat Candida Diet*, but as with any ingredient,

cut them out if you suspect they are not good for your particular metabolism and digestive weakness.

Grains

The balance between proteins and carbohydrates is very
important, and we have referred to this earlier in Chapter 6.
Unfortunately some people with candida cannot tolerate any
grains, although with long-term treatment that situation can
usually be reversed. Millet, brown rice, and quinoa (pro-
nounced keenwa) are the most used grains in our recipes.
Quinoa is a new grain from South America which contains
more protein than any other grain, and is easy to digest. You
could also try buckwheat. Despite its name it is not a wheat.

Beans and pulses

These are a wonderful source of protein when combined with
grains. Some are more easily digested than others. If you have a
problem soak for two days, so that they are almost sprouting,
replace the water and cook with a strip of kombu (a sea vegetable). Apart from lentils and various beans, try orange and
green split peas in soups, with added cumin for flavour and
interest. Tinned pulses can be used for emergencies and quick
cooking, but rinse before use, and buy brands which have no
sugar added.

Alternatives to cow's milk

Fewer people are sensitive to sheep's milk, and it has a softer
taste than goats' milk. Sheep's milk freezes well, but goats' milk
is probably easier to find. Other 'milks' come from grains, such
as rice milk (Rice Dream) and oat milk. Soya milk is sometimes
tolerated and sometimes not. We have not used it because many
dislike the taste, and we are wary about genetically engineered
soya which may now be found in all non-organic soya prod-

ucts. However, you may find it an acceptable milk to substitute for some of the others.

Whatever you read about candida, there is bound to be a different view, and alternative 'rules', especially when it comes to food. Our view is that the best results can be gained by combining the healing quality of foods with supplements as appropriate to avoid unnecersarily limited dietary choices.

By this means you are healing the gut wall, and at the same time paying attention to fine-tuning your digestion. Some books say 'no carrots' and some say 'yes to mushrooms'. Others say, like this, 'no wheat' but 'yes' to rye and oats, which also contain gluten. Whatever the 'line', take it on board only in relation to *your* responses and reactions. You are the best person to judge. As you get used to 'listening' to your body, and paying attention to its reactions, you will be better able to pinpoint what may have caused some of your symptoms. Whatever happens though, don't blame food all the time. The stresses in our lives play a large part too, and making changes, apart from food, is sometimes part of the recovery process.

Chapter Nine

The *Beat Candida Diet*

After diagnosis, you will need to decide how quickly you are going to be able to start the programme and to what extent you will need to adapt your normal diet. If you eat a high propor-tion of convenience foods, saturated fats, sugar, and stimulants such as coffee, it may be sensible to make changes slowly over time, before plunging headlong into the total anti-candida programme. This is because making so many changes at once is difficult.

On the other hand you may be so ill that you will do any-thing to get better quickly. A lot depends on your tempera-ment, your motivation, and the level of support others are willing to give you. For those of you horrified at the prospect of living without bread, or sugar, we provide day-to-day guide-lines on how to make basic changes before moving on to the specific programme outlined in Chapter 5, and tips on how to deal with cravings.

If your diet is already based on many of the principles of the anti-candida diet, and you are familiar with many of the foods, you will find it easier to start straight away. For most, however, there are three stages to go through on the diet:

● *Stage 1:* The 2 Week Action Plan
  This could take longer than 2 weeks if you want it to. It is the adjustment phase. You will be introduced to new ingredients, new eating principles, and will gradually adapt to doing without the foods which exacerbate your condi-tion.

- *Stage 2:* The Candida Control Programme
  This is the most rigorous phase of the diet, based on the principles of food combining. For a clear explanation of how and why you should keep starch and protein foods separate see page 71. Use only those recipes marked ✓ or FC (Food Combining) for this phase. It could take up to 3 months to be clear of candida overgrowth, and longer if you have chronic candida.

- *Stage 3:* The Maintenance Diet
  At this point you should be clear of symptoms and be able to begin to reintroduce certain foods. See page 112.

Shopping List

Before you start the programme we provide you with a shopping list and advice on where to buy ingredients. Your budget may be stretched for a time while you are buying supplements. You will need, or should consider:

For yourself:
- bristle brush for dry skin brushing from health food shops or via mail order
- plant-based digestive enzymes
- a good yeast-free multi-vitamin and mineral combination

For the kitchen:
- a water filter or under the sink unit
- a stainless steel collapsible steamer (Bamboo ones could harbour bacteria)
- a wok for quick cooking with stir-frying
- a salad spinner
- hard brush for scrubbing organic vegetables
- ginger grater
- wide-topped flask for transporting hot food
- plastic or glass containers for food storage
- food processor and/or liquidiser

- coffee grinder especially for spices
- juicer
- pressure cooker for well cooked grains and ease of digestion.

We have not added to the list a microwave. However, if you already have one, there is nothing wrong in resorting to using them in emergencies. They may be useful for heating up food, or defrosting. Try not to cook all your food this way however, and remember not to store your vitamins and minerals on top of microwaves, they will be affected by radiation. A freezer is useful for making several batches of food at once, for quick snacks and meals.

Ingredients:

These are some of the stand-by foods you will need to have at home in order to follow our recipes for candida control. If you need to stagger your purchases go for the starred items★ first. They are often cheaper in health food shops than supermarkets, because they are sold in larger quantities or are unbranded goods.

- wheatfree tamari (Bragg or Soji)
- cold pressed virgin olive oil in opaque bottles to keep out the light★
- unfiltered organic cider vinegar in large opaque bottles to keep out the light★
- alfalfa seeds★
- yeastfree vegetable stock
- sea-salt
- organic porridge oats★
- organic jumbo oats
- organic Rice flakes★
- rice syrup (for the first two weeks only)
- quinoa★
- organic Millet★
- organic brown rice★

- organic maize flour
- organic potato flour
- coconut block★ or coconut milk
- sea vegetables – kombu, nori (if you need to watch your spending buy only one variety at a time)
- organic sunflower seeds★ (you will need large amounts of these for snacks as well as cooking)
- unhulled sesame seeds★
- organic pumpkin seeds★
- tahini (sesame paste, available in large tubs in health food shops)
- herbal teas – peppermint, camomile, rooibosch, pau d'arco, ginger
- oat milk
- fresh almonds★ (there is a higher turnover in well-used health food shops)
- Organic linseeds and/or best quality linseed oil in dark bottles★
- cumin seeds
- coriander seeds
- black mustard seeds
- turmeric
- cayenne pepper
- root ginger★
- soft goat's cheese★
- goat's milk
- sheep's milk
- live goat's and sheep's yoghurt★
- Russian rye bread★ (yeast-free. Can be ordered via mail order if not readily available.)
- Sprouted rye bread (yeast-free)★
- Non-malted Ryvita
- oat cakes (wheatfree)
- rice cakes
- Vitaquell margarine or any unhydrogenated margarine
- organic eggs★ (not the same as free-range)

- organic pulses such as lentils, split peas, mung beans, butter-beans, chickpeas, white beans★
- Cans of tuna, sardines, chickpeas (for quick curries and hummus), artichoke hearts (for dips and salads), coconut milk (the block is more economical)

Tips for storage

It is best to transfer herbs and spices bought from health food shops in plastic bags to glass jars. Plastic takes away the taste in time. Herbs and spices are best stored out of the light.

If you have a problem fitting your new foods in your cupboard invest in small cheap baskets to hold your packets on the work surface. Keeping new staples visible is a good idea at this stage. You will be reminded of them, and inspired to use them.

Preparing the kitchen

- Take time before you start Stage 1 to defrost and clean out the fridge, and throw away any limp, bruised or decaying food. It is vital for your new diet that you do not eat any food showing signs of decay or mould.
- Throw in the bin any out of date spices, seeds and nuts.
- Discard old oils and all margarines, except Vitaquell. You will be doing your family a favour, as well as yourself. Substitute with unsalted butter, if possible.
- Give away or throw away all your wheat-based breads, biscuits, cakes and snacks. Take heart that over the weeks your need for sugar, cakes and biscuits will diminish.

Ready to start

As a way of easing you into the programme try each day to do the following:

- Wake up and drink a glass of lemon water – a slice of lemon covered with cold water, and topped up with hot water. This is detoxifying and good for the peristaltic action of the colon. Add crushed root ginger too.

- Dry skin brush before your shower or bath.
- Remember to drink plenty of filtered or bottled water over and above any hot drinks you consume.
- Never miss breakfast. If you find breakfast hard to eat, and eat only fruit, eat half a grapefruit, or a grated apple and yoghurt. Have a snack ready to eat later when you are hungry. In Stage 2 you may need to cut down on fruit for a while.
- Eat little and often. Follow our snacks guide, as well as meal plans.
- Plan to eat your main meal of the day at lunch time and have a light meal at night instead. This is because you should eat main evening meals before eight in the evening, to allow time to digest before going to bed.

Stage 1: The 2-Week Action Plan

This stage gradually introduces you to some of the principles underlying candida control. We do not assume that you will be able to follow all of the principles in Chapter 6 straight away, but the choice is there for you to take at whatever pace you feel comfortable with. For example, you may decide to increase your ratio of vegetables to animal protein from day one, or you may do it gradually over several weeks. You can stay in your comfort zone, if that is what you need, by adding potatoes or rice, or other carbohydrates when eating protein. This will stop in Stage 2.

Remember you are having to let go of easy options based on routine and habit. Be kind to yourself in these early days, and follow your intuition about the pace of change you can manage, especially if you have others to cook for who have no intention of changing their diets. (It is amazing how many do adapt, once they are presented with more food choices, and an opportunity to try new approaches to cooking.)

At this stage we recommend you get all the help you can to improve your digestion by investing in some digestive enzymes to give yourself a boost. Then when you begin Stage 2, cut down the enzymes as your body becomes better able to do the job itself.

Because this programme is designed to allow you to move at whatever pace suits your circumstances, you may choose to start by following recommendations for only one meal per day, say breakfasts. This is often a hurried and fraught meal, and is one that many candida sufferers find the most difficult.

After a couple of weeks, you may wish to tackle evening meals. By this time you will have moved beyond the anxiety of not knowing how to cope at all. Make it easy for yourself – some of your lunches in the two week action plan could be leftovers from the night before, as long as you are not hyper-sensitive to mould. If you need your food to be portable, re-heated food can be transported in a wide-topped flask. This cuts down on the difficulty of planning for packed lunches, and the risk of being caught out with no substitutes, such as rye bread or fresh salads.

You may find it difficult to make changes in how you eat and prepare food, when you are feeling ill and lacking in energy. This is why we lead you into the *Beat Candida Diet* slowly, so that when you are eventually ready to move to Stage 2, (under the care of a practitioner to give support) you are more pre-pared for the toxic effects of 'die-off' in the early stages of taking anti-fungal supplements.

Day 1

Start on a day in which you have plenty of time to do the groundwork. Your main task today is to find where to buy some of the foods which are going to help you on the *Beat Candida Diet*. This is not a day for experimenting with new ways of eating – eat your normal diet while you get ready to put the diet into practice. Limit your coffee and tea intake however. Try the Chinese Kemun tea without milk as a half-way measure. It contains very little tannin. Some come infused with mango or passion flowers and are very refreshing.

You will need to:
- Investigate your local health food shop – try some of the independent ones for a committed approach to food quality and choice.
- Find the whereabouts of local organic suppliers, including your supermarket
- Ring the Soil Association for a list of local box fruit and vegetable schemes.
- Do you have any local farms with organic produce, willing to sell at the farm gate?

Day 2

Breakfast
Substitute herbal teas for coffee and tea.
Apart from their benefits, herbal teas are not taken with milk, so giving up dairy products is easier this way.
Rye bread toast with butter and sugarless jam
or
Porridge with banana and cinnamon
(Later you will need to eat fruit separately from all other foods, to eliminate fermentation in the stomach after eating fruit.)

Lunch
Baked organic potato and Winter Coleslaw with Mayonnaise

Supper
Mixed Vegetable Curry with brown rice
or
Marinated Lamb Kebabs
Plain live yoghurt with sliced kiwi fruit
(Kiwi fruit is a sour fruit, and less of a problem for most than other sweeter fruits.)

Get to bed early – you may need to rest if your body is missing caffeine.

Snacks
- Apples, bananas, pears, pawpaw, kiwis, avocado (get used to having only two pieces of fruit a day). NO grapes, melons, oranges or soft fruit. ● Hummus with carrot and celery sticks ● oat cakes ● ryvita ● any pâté made with mashed pulses and seasonings ● tinned artichoke hearts (whizzed in blender with olive oil and garlic for a dip) ● tamari seeds ● yoghurt and roasted sunflower seeds ● avocado on rye bread ● soft goat's cheese with vegetable sticks.

Day 3

Breakfast
Scrambled Egg Mexican Style with rice cakes
(Eggs cooked with vegetables provide a more balanced meal than on their own, but if red pepper and garlic are too much at this time of day, just go for fried onion and chopped tomato.)

Lunch
Tuna pâté and Ryvita with cucumber slices
or
left-over Vegetable Curry

Supper
Puy Lentils and Courgettes
or

Grilled chicken or fish
Serve with large helping of cauliflower with coriander and sunflower seeds, and carrots and sesame seeds with sesame oil. Add
to this some stir-fried greens with tamari, garlic and ginger.
(Broccoli tops are delicious, as are spring greens.)

Evening: Begin sprouting alfalfa seeds

Day 4

Rinse the sprouts, and dry roast some seeds for snacks in the day.

Breakfast
Rice porridge and 1 teaspoon rice syrup or ¼ banana

Lunch
Onion Soup with Spinach and Ginger
or
Leftovers from last night blended into a soup.

Early evening
Ginger tea. Add half a teaspoon of rice syrup if you are unused
to the taste. (At Stage 2, rice syrup will be phased out.)

Supper
Tuna, Broccoli and Celeriac Casserole, and another green vegetable.
or
Red Peppers Stuffed with Rice and Almonds

Evening: Rinse the sprouts. Soak some almonds

Day 5

Rinse the sprouts.

Breakfast
Muesli with grated apple, seeds and soaked almonds

Lunch
Quinoa Salad tabbouleh style

Mid-afternoon
Warming ginger tea, this time sweetened with apple juice. (Fruit juice is not allowed at Stage 2 because of its quick acting sugars.)

Supper
Millet, courgettes, green beans and thyme risotto with soft goat's cheese, and stir fried carrots and greens.

Evening: Soak mung beans. Rinse sprouts. Soak oats in boiling water and place in oven overnight.

Day 6

Rinse sprouts.

Breakfast
Savoury Vegetable Pancakes
or
No-Sweat Porridge

Lunch
Chickpea and Carrot Soup
or
Leftovers of Millet Risotto whizzed in blender with extra stock to make a soup, with added sprouted almonds and fresh garlic.

Supper
Avocado and Green Pea Guacomole Dip with corn chips
Fish in a Parcel with Nutty Vegetable Shreds
Potato Rosti and Ginger Spinach

Evening: Rinse mung beans

Drinks
- herbal teas – rooibosch, peppermint, camomile, taheebo, pau d'arco
- bottled water
- ginger tea
- lemon water
- Keemun tea
- most coffee substitutes are malted, and need to be avoided in Stage 2. Later on try Barley Cup or Yannoh.

Day 7

Marinate organic chicken

Breakfast
Toasted rye bread with tahini or soaked muesli and yoghurt

Lunch
Marinated Roast Chicken with Garlic and Mustard Seeds
Baked Spanish Onions with Goat's Cheese
Asparagus with Tarragon and Lemon
Potato with olive oil, and chives

Supper
Sprouted Mung Bean, Celery and Green Bean Soup

Evening: Soak linseeds in water

Day 8

Breakfast
Swallow linseeds whole with plenty of water. (If you wish, chew a few to release their GLA. Whole seeds are best for ensuring regular bowel movements.)
Organic Rice Puffs with oatmilk and almonds

Lunch
Green Soup and Cheesy Muffins with Celariac, Carrot and Mayonnaise Salad

Supper
Stir-fried Cabbage with Lime and Coconut, with chicken from the day before.
Carrots and ginger
or
Spicy Aubergine and Potato Crust.

Evening: Soak sunflower seeds

Day 9

Rinse sunflower seeds

Breakfast
Sprouted rye bread with mashed avocado and lemon

Lunch
Baked Potato and Winter Coleslaw with Sea Vegetables, Mustard and Lemon and alfalfa sprouts.

Supper
Carrot, Broccoli and Parsnip Korma with brown rice and Curried Lentil Gravy (dahl)

Evening: Rinse sunflower seeds

Day 10

Rinse sunflower seeds
Breakfast
Rice Porridge with cardamom and banana

Lunch
Hard-boiled egg, watercress, and alfalfa sprouts, with Grated

Carrot and Sesame Seeds. Eat with oat cakes, rye bread or rice cakes.

Supper
Hurdy Gurdy Vegetable Soup
Fresh Sardine Crackers and stir-fried leeks

Evening: Rinse sunflower seeds

Day 11

Breakfast
Soaked sunflower seeds, live yoghurt and grated apple with optional muesli

Lunch
Savoury Nutty Seed Cakes and tomato and avocado salad

Supper
Roasted Vegetable Quinoa

Evening: Soak linseeds in water

Day 12

Breakfast
Swallow linseeds
Scrambled Egg: Mexican Style

Lunch
New Potato and Sunflower Seed Salad with Celery, Cucumber and Red Onion Salsa

Supper
Thai Fish-cakes with Coriander, with Mange-tout, Asparagus and Spring onion, Stir-fry

Evening: Soak sea vegetables. Soak oats in boiling water and place in oven overnight.

Day 13

Breakfast
No-sweat porridge

Lunch
Hummus, made with tinned rinsed chickpeas, with vegetable sticks and rye bread.

Supper
Poached Salmon with Herbs, with Sea Vegetable and Grated Courgette Stir-fry

Evening: Soak the butterbeans and almonds for the next day.

Day 14

Breakfast
Dry-roasted porridge with nutmeg and live yoghurt (Plus optional rice syrup, soon to be dropped.)

Lunch
Pheasant Casserole with Celery and Baby Onions, Brussels sprouts and Colcannon
or
Butterbean, Aubergine and Celeriac purée, with vegetable pancakes

Supper
Mixed Onion Soup with cabbage parcels

> ## Quick ideas for lunch
> - Hummus whizzed up using a tin of chick-peas eaten with carrot sticks
> - Lettuce leaves stuffed with slices of avocado, tomatoes, olives and basil with olive oil
> - Lettuce leaves stuffed with coleslaw and mayonnaise
> - Take-away Japanese sushi (Nori seaweed wrapped round rice and vegetables.) Avoid those with pickles
> - Yoghurt and sunflower seeds
> - Baked onion, instead of the usual baked potato, with goat's cheese
> - Soup

After this gradual introduction, over a number of weeks, you should be used to soaking the linseeds, making tamari seeds for snacks, and sprouting. The regular morning routine of lemon water and skin brushing should become automatic. Regular exercise, such as brisk walking, is also important. If it is hard to get out, invest in a rebounder, (a mini-trampoline). This is an excellent form of exercise for the lymphatics.

Stage 2: The Candida Control Programme

As you move into the Candida Control Programme you may need to limit your fruit intake, to two pieces a day. (Read *Fit for Life* for a detailed explanation of why fruit should be eaten separately from other food in order to cut out fermentation.) Although rice syrup and sugarless jam are not allowed on Stage 1, you may be able to tolerate rice syrup, in small amounts. The main difference in Stage 2 is that we recommend you follow food combining rules from now on. Recipes which are not marked FC (Food Combining) should be put aside for occasional use during Stage 3 the maintenance stage, after recovery.

As you start to take probiotics and antifungal supplements (see pages 54–7), you may experience your symptoms worse than before. If this happens just concentrate on doing quick and simple meals for a week or so, such as stir-fries, grains and soups.

During Stage 2 the practitioner's role is crucial. Working on many levels, the practitioner should monitor progress, and ensure that your attitude to the diet is not so rigid that fear or failure is the predominant motivating factor. Fear does not help the digestive process and could play a part in perpetuating the Candida problem. For some, the rigidity of the diet seems to exacerbate a controlling personality trait that needs to be loosened up. For healing to occur you need to be open to change and less judgemental. Rigidity does not allow for adaptation and free interpretation of the 'rules' in line with your own body's needs. In time you will learn to recognise your own response to certain foods and how those responses change over time, thereby allowing more choice, or necessitating temporary restrictions according to your personal needs. After three months or so you should test your reaction to yeast based foods, to assess tolerance.

Stage 3: The Maintenance Diet

Once you have recovered you will enter the maintenance phase At this stage you will find that you will be able to extend your food choices, and digest more complex meals. Take care to follow the supplements guidelines for maintenance in chapter 5, and watch out for any flare up symptoms. If this happens, revert to the diet in Stage 2 and assess the need for anti-fungals or probiotics. Try and assess if there is any reason for the flare-up which may be related to avoidable stresses in your life.

Recovery time

Of the many people with candida problems who we talk to each year, it is those who accept the challenge of the candida diet, and relish the prospect of cooking appetising and nutritious meals, who get better the soonest. Those who react with

'I can't' and 'I've tried everything' are not helping their recovery. Honouring the process of buying food, cooking food , and eating food is absolutely essential for long-term recovery.

With the advent of new and more effective supplements for candida you should be heartened to know that most people with mild to average candida problems recover within six months, depending how committed they are to the programme. Others, who have been ill for longer, may take longer, particularly if candida is complicated by CFS or ME. Whatever the extent of your individual problem, we hope that most of the recipes in this book have something for everyone. What better way to recover, than to eat not just for 'health' but also for pleasure!

Eating out

- Be cautious of open salad bars and raw food, especially in fast food chains, because of dressings and toppings, and problems of oxidation from food left lying around.
- Choose fresh fish first. Ask for simple combinations, such as grilling without sauces. Or choose a well cooked omelette with herbs or vegetables
- Select Oriental, Indian or Mexican restaurants – culturally their cuisine fits the diet better than European ways of cooking. If you eat at Greek, or Middle Eastern restaurants – think 'Hummus, lamb, and mezze'. Watch out for tabbouleh and couscous – wheat!
- Indian breads are made from low-gluten flour and are flat and unleavened – some people can tolerate this on the *Beat Candida Diet*.
- Healthfood and vegetarian restaurants can be difficult in the UK because traditionally they use so much wheat and cheese – pizza and pasta, thickened soups and stews with wheat, and tempting crumbles, quiches and tarts – definitely out of the question during Stage 2.
- If possible avoid all fast-food chains, motorway service stations and food at most pubs (except the new 'food conscious'

ones). Their food is chemically compromised, usually prepared elsewhere, full of fats and bulked up with wheat. Staff
will have no idea what ingredient went into which dish
because they are hired to serve the food, not to prepare it.

- Ring the restaurant in advance if you have not been to it
  before, to check what you could have from the menu. Seek
  out family businesses who are more inclined to care.

- It is a good idea to thank helpful staff, chefs and waiters, and
  say you will recommend friends with similar problems to
  visit. This will encourage the restaurant to provide a variety
  of foods and information.

- Don't be shy about talking to friends about your dietary
  requirements if you are invited out to eat. If they seem worried about being able to meet your needs, suggest that you
  take your own substitute – or lend them this book!

- Take your herbal teas, ginger, digestive enzymes, Ryvita and
  oat cakes with you wherever you go.

- When travelling, take a picnic – buy a heating element for
  the car cigarette lighter to heat up drinks and soups, or take
  a thermos.

Part III

The *Beat Candida Diet* Recipes

- All recipes are suitable for Stages 1 and 3 of the Beat Candida Diet.
- Use only those Food Combining recipes marked ✓ at Stage 2.
- Some recipes cross-reference to others in the book. For a full recipe listing, see the index.
- For ease of reference recipes are marked GLUTENFREE, DAIRYFREE, EGGFREE, YEASTFREE, FOOD COMBINING (FC) so you can monitor your own dietary needs

When using these recipes it is useful to familiarise yourself with the text beforehand in order to understand some of the basic principles of the diet. The recipes are intended as a base on which to adapt and build to your preferences and needs. Optional ingredients such as chillies, should be used with caution because they may not agree with you. Taking them out will not alter the recipe too much.

- Organic vegetables These should be used wherever possible. They should not be peeled because most of the vitamin content is under the skin. However, if you have to use non-organic root vegetables we recommend you do peel them because of high levels of organo-phosphates.
- Salt In many recipes no salt has been listed in the ingredients because the spices used usually compensate for salt. But if you find that you require extra seasoning then add to your taste. Use sea-salt in preference to other salts because it has valuable trace elements.
- Rice When cooking rice you can either use long or short grain rice. Short grain rice cooks to a creamier texture, which is why it is suitable for risottos. Because of this it is easier to digest. Do not use white rice on the diet because it is nutritionally deficient, and is a refined carboydrate.
- Measurements: Where we refer to 'cups' you may use the same sized cup measure or tea-cup all the time, so that proportions stay the same.

Staple recipes

Soaked Linseeds ✓

GLUTENFREE, DAIRYFREE, EGGFREE, YEASTFREE, FC

Place 1 dsp linseeds in a glass and cover with water. Soak overnight and swallow whole before breakfast, with plenty of liquid.

Sea Vegetable Seasoning ✓

GLUTENFREE, DAIRYFREE, EGGFREE, YEASTFREE, FC

Place ½oz (15g) of mixed sea vegetable flakes in a coffee grinder and grind until reduced to smaller flakes. Store in a glass jar in the fridge and add to all the recipes in the *Beat Candida Diet* which call for Sea Vegetable Seasoning.

Ginger Tea ✓

serves 1

GLUTENFREE, DAIRYFREE, EGGFREE, YEASTFREE, FC

Take a knob of root ginger about half the size of your thumb and peel with a knife or vegetable peeler. Grate the ginger on the coarse side of a cheese grater, place in a saucepan and simmer for 10–15 minutes. Allow it to cool before drinking.

The grated ginger can be steeped several times during the day without losing its strength.

Sprouting Alfalfa ✓

GLUTENFREE, DAIRYFREE, EGGFREE, YEASTFREE, FC

**2 tbsp alfalfa seeds
large jam jar
rubber band for lid
muslin square**

Wash the seeds, place in the jam jar and cover with water.

Cover with a lid and secure with the rubber band. Leave overnight in a warm room.

The next morning pour off the excess water through the muslin.

Continue to rinse the seeds morning and night for 4-5 days, or until the seeds have long delicate white sprouts massed together like a bird's nest. When fully sprouted, store in the fridge for up to 3 days.

Eat in handfuls with almonds, sunflower or pumpkin seeds, or in a salad. Sprouts can also be added to soups, stews and stir-fries; as a garnish as they need no cooking.

Ghee ✓

GLUTENFREE, DAIRYFREE (SEE NOTE),
EGGFREE, YEASTFREE, FC

Ghee is the Indian version of clarified butter, where cooking removes the milk solids from the oil. Milk solids increase mucous, and non-organic butter may also contain hormones or antibodies. Best of all, clarified butter contains no lactose, so it is ideal for use in frying on the *Beat Candida Diet*.

Melt the butter over low heat. As the fat liquefies the milk proteins will rise to the surface. Turn off the heat and allow the proteins to sink to the bottom. Carefully pour off the oil (through muslin or cheesecloth is best) into a glass container (preferably coloured), leaving behind the white proteins which can be discarded.

Ghee keeps well and cooks well as a partner to olive oil – half ghee, half olive oil.

Cook' note
Ghee is usually safe to use on a dairyfree diet as the milk proteins have been discarded.

Almond Milk   ✓

serves 1

GLUTENFREE, DAIRYFREE, EGGFREE, YEASTFREE, FC

---

4 tbsp almonds (shelled)
I cup (measuring or teacup) water

Shell the almonds by placing in boiling water for 1 minute. Slip off the skins after rinsing under cold water. Blend the almonds and water until white and smooth. Drink straight away for breakfast or store for up to 3 days in the fridge.

Add a banana when blending on Stage 1 and 3 of the *Beat Candida Diet* and/or cinnamon or nutmeg.

Cooks's note
An excellent source of protein and calcium.

Breakfasts

Morning Vegetable Juice ✓

serves 1

GLUTENFREE, DAIRYFREE, EGGFREE, YEASTFREE, FC

4 celery sticks, chopped
2 carrots, peeled and chopped
6 sprigs of parsley
6 sprigs of watercress

Juice all the ingredients and drink immediately.

To balance the flavour, add 1 tbsp cider vinegar or a light sprinkling of cayenne pepper or Sea Vegetable Seasoning, to make up the right taste for you.

Cook's note
Juices must be fresh to be effective and should be consumed first thing in the morning or as a revitaliser taken without food at any time of the day.

Jeremy's Rice Porridge ✓

serves 1

GLUTENFREE, DAIRYFREE, EGGFREE, YEASTFREE, FC

I cup rice flakes
2 cups of water

Optional:
Seeds from three cardomon pods
I tsp Tahini
knob of ghee
¼ banana sliced
or
in Stage I (only)
I teaspoon rice syrup

This recipe was given to us by Jeremy Jones, who invented it to use as a 'summer porridge'.

Combine the flakes, liquid and cardomon seeds, stirring frequently, and cook over a low heat for 5 minutes. Add tahini and ghee for additional smothness and flavour. Cut out the ghee if you do not want it to be too rich.

Oat Porridge ✓

serves 1

GLUTENFREE, DAIRYFREE, EGGFREE, YEASTFREE, FC

I cup oats
2 cups of water

Optional:
yoghurt
banana
nutmeg
rice syrup (Stage I only)

We recommend you use organic rolled or pinhead oats for this porridge. Most health-food stores sell rolled oats in large amounts, which makes it cheaper than prepared oats in cardboard boxes.

Soak the oats overnight, or alternatively, dry roast before adding water to cook to cut down on cooking time. When you are not able to sweeten in the normal way, this gives extra flavour and interest, especially if you add yoghurt, nutmeg and banana (Stages 1 and 3 only) once the porridge is cooked.

Heat the porridge gently, after soaking all night, stirring most of the time, until creamy and smooth. Serve with optional additions.

No-sweat (no saucepan) Porridge ✓

serves 1

GLUTENFREE, DAIRYFREE, EGGFREE, YEASTFREE, FC

Place I cup of oats in 4 cups of boiling water in a heatproof dish or bowl the night before. Leave covered in a very low oven to be ready in the morning. The ultimate convenience food and deliciously creamy.

Cook's note

To dry roast oats: place unsoaked oats in the bottom of a saucepan, and over a gentle heat stir them for a minute or two until they start to go crisp and brown at the edges. Slowly add the water and cook in the normal way.

Millet porridge can also be made to ring the changes.

Muesli   ✓

serves 1

GLUTENFREE, DAIRYFREE, EGGFREE, YEASTFREE, FC

Do not use commercial varieties of muesli which are sweetened. If you buy a made-up sugar-free muesli base from a
health food shop buy one without raisins or nuts. If you wish to
add nuts they must be freshly shelled. Homemade muesli can be
made with a variety of grains – oats, millet flakes, brown rice
flakes, and barley flakes. If you want it to be entirely gluten-free
leave out the barley. Finding the balance that you like is important. Once again, health food shops will have these ingredients.

Optional extras:
Sprouted almonds, flaked coconut, grated apple

Add each day:
Freshly ground linseeds
Freshly ground sunflower seeds
Freshly ground sesame seeds
Whole pumpkin seeds

Option:
Soak overnight to bring out the natural sweetness of the grains.

Stage 1:
Soak in apple juice, with a few raisins

Breakfasts

Jeremy's Rice porridge	Jumbo oats with seeds
Soaked oat porridge	Almond milk with banana
Dry-roasted porridge	Scrambled eggs Mexican style
No-sweat porridge	Toasted rye bread
Millet porridge	Organic Rice Puffs
Muesli	

Eggs

Eggs Florentine with Sea Vegetable Seasoning

serves 2

GLUTENFREE, DAIRYFREE, YEASTFREE, NO ADDED SUGAR

**450 g/1 lb fresh cooked spinach, or 225 g/8 oz frozen spinach,
thawed and drained of moisture
nutmeg and Sea Vegetable Seasoning
black pepper
2 organic or free range eggs
40 g/1 1/2 oz butter, ghee, margarine or olive oil
4 spring onions, 1 leek or 1/2 onion, chopped
25 g/1 oz cornflour, arrowroot, kombu
275 ml/10 fl oz stock
1 tsp Bragg or other wheatfree, yeastfree tamari**

Preheat the oven to 190°C/375°F/Gas Mark 5.

Grease a small ovenproof dish. Make sure the cooked spinach is as 'dry' as possible by pushing it down in a sieve or colander with a potato masher or back of a wooden spoon. Arrange the spinach on the base of the dish. Season with nutmeg, some sea vegetable seasoning (you don't need salt – it's in the seasoning) and black pepper.

Make a sauce by melting or heating the chosen fat or oil in a pan and sautéing the chosen onion or leek until transparent.

Slake the cornflour, arrowroot or kombu with a *little* cool stock in a cup. Return this to the rest of the stock and mix well. Add to the onion mixture in the pan, stir well and heat until thickened and glossy. Add the Bragg or other tamari and beat again.

Make 2 depressions in the spinach and gently break an egg into each one. Pour the sauce over the contents of the dish, to cover them completely, and bake for 10–15 minutes, or until the eggs are set.

For a treat, dot with soft goat's cheese before baking.

Scrambled Egg Mexican Style   ✓

serves 1

GLUTENFREE, DAIRYFREE, YEASTFREE, FC

---

1 tsp ghee or olive oil
1 spring onion, chopped
1 small garlic clove, sliced
1 small piece of red pepper, chopped
1 small tomato, chopped (optional)
1 organic egg, beaten
2 sprigs of coriander or parsley, chopped

Heat the ghee or oil in a pan. Add the spring onion, garlic, pepper and tomato if using, and fry for 2 minutes over low heat , stirring constantly. Add the beaten egg and continue cooking and stirring until the egg has scrambled. If you use an organic egg it's fine to have a 'wet' scramble, but if using non-organic egg make sure the egg has cooked to a 'dry' scramble.

Serve sprinkled with fresh coriander or chopped parsley.

For a spicier, hotter mixture, add a pinch of cayenne pepper or small piece of chopped green chilli to the vegetables when cooking.

Cook's note
Stage 1 and 3
Serve on rye bread or rye toast.
This mixture is excellent cold on rice or oat cakes, or as a sandwich mixture.

Egg Mayonnaise on Rye Bread

serves 1

WHEATFREE, DAIRYFREE, YEASTFREE

**1 hard-boiled organic egg (boiled for 7 minutes
then plunge into cold running water)
1 spring onion, finely chopped
1 tbsp Mayonnaise (see page 132)
1 tsp lemon or lime juice
1 tsp grated lemon or lime rind
2 very thin slices of rye or glutenfree bread
4 slices of cucumber
black pepper**

Tap the egg several times on the side of the sink and peel off the shell. Chop well and mix with the spring onion, mayonnaise, lemon juice and rind. Spread thinly on the bread and garnish with cucumber slices and several grinds of black pepper.

Well-scrambled eggs could be used instead of egg mayonnaise.

Cook's Note
To take this in a lunch box, roll the bread up as if making asparagus rolls, packing the cucumber separately. Or, since glutenfree bread is difficult to roll, take the ingredients separately and assemble when you're ready to eat.

Alternatively, substitute asparagus tips for the egg mayonnaise and roll up carefully.

Spanish Omelette   ✓

serves 4

GLUTENFREE, DAIRYFREE, YEASTFREE, FC

A quantity of left-over cooked vegetables (but not potato or parsnip), or 225g/8oz fresh vegetables, carrots, leeks, broccoli, cabbage, Brussels sprouts, peeled
1–2 tbsp mixed ghee and olive oil
1 medium onion, chopped
3 garlic cloves, sliced
1 red pepper, chopped
6 organic eggs, beaten
2 tbsp mixed chopped fresh herbs – parsley, coriander, oregano, chives, or 1 tbsp mixed dried herbs
50 g/2 oz soft goat's cheese (optional)

Chop the cooked vegetables into even-sized pieces. If using fresh vegetables, cut into small pieces and blanch in boiling water for 4 minutes.

Melt the ghee and olive oil in a large frying pan and sauté the onion, garlic and chopped red pepper until the onion is translucent. Add the mixed vegetables and sauté for a further 3 minutes, stirring constantly. Pour on the beaten eggs , add the herbs and stir for a minute to mix the eggs into the vegetables. Reduce the heat and let the omelette set and cook underneath.

If using goat's cheese, dot it over the surface of the omelette just before serving to allow the heat to melt the cheese.

Slide the omelette on to a large dish with the help of a fish slice, and divide into portions.

Serve with a green salad.

Coriander and Coconut Egg Curry ✓

serves 4

GLUTENFREE, DAIRYFREE, YEASTFREE, FC

---

3 garlic cloves, roughly chopped
50g/2oz creamed coconut from a block
I dsp coriander seeds
I tsp mustard seeds
I tsp curry powder
2 tbsp ghee
2 large onions, finely chopped
150ml/5 fl oz live plain yoghurt
¼ mild green chilli, finely chopped (use rubber gloves)
I tbsp lemon juice
black pepper
2 tbsp chopped coriander
4 hard boiled organic eggs (boiled for 7 minutes,
then plunged into cold running water)

Using a coffee grinder or blender, process the garlic, coriander and mustard seeds and curry powder until finely ground.

Heat the ghee in a large frying pan and fry the onions until golden. Using a slotted spoon, remove the onions mix with the yoghurt.

Add the spice mixture to the ghee and fry for 3 minutes, stirring constantly. Stir in the yoghurt mixture and creamed coconut and simmer, until the coconut has dissolved, about for 30 mins. Add the green chilli, lemon juice, several turns of black pepper and the coriander to the mixture, and turn off the heat.

Shell the eggs and cut in half. Pour the curry sauce over the eggs and serve with a vegetable such as leeks.

Cook's notes
Serving with rice will break the food combining rules – not recommended on Stage 2.

Stocks, sauces and dressings

Vegetable Stock ✓

makes 1.75 litres, 3 pints

GLUTENFREE, DAIRYFREE, EGGFREE, YEASTFREE, FC

**2 large onions, sliced
6 carrots, peeled and sliced
I head of celery, chopped
strip of lemon peel
small strip of root ginger
I garlic clove
bunch of herbs – parsley, thyme, oregano
3.4l/⅙ pts water**

Put all the ingredients into a very large saucepan. Bring to the boil and simmer for 25 minutes. Strain or, if using a pressure cooker, reduce the amount of water to the maximum allowed for your type of cooker, bring to pressure and steam for 15 minutes. Strain. Use immediately to make other recipes or freeze in cartons until required.

The vegetables used in making the stock may become part of the next soup recipe by processing till smooth in a processor or blender and adding to 900ml/1½ pints of the vegetable stock.

Herb Dressing   ✓

GLUTENFREE, DAIRYFREE, EGGFREE, YEASTFREE, FC

---

100 ml/4 fl oz cider vinegar
100 ml/4 fl oz lemon juice
350 ml/12 fl oz water
1 tbsp. crushed garlic
3 tbsp grain mustard
2 tbsp finely chopped parsley
2 tsp sea salt
1/8 tsp pepper
2 tbsp finely chopped red pepper
1/4 tsp each dried oregano, basil and thyme
1 tsp agar agar flakes

In a food processor or blender, blend all the ingredients except the agar agar flakes. Add the flakes and blend again for 1 minute to thicken.

Refrigerate in a screw-top jar and use within 2 weeks to dress any salad, or vegetables like shredded cabbage, leeks or broccoli.

Garlic and Cardamom Dressing   ✓

GLUTENFREE, DAIRYFREE, EGGFREE, YEASTFREE
(IF USING YEASTFREE TAMARI), FC

---

1 crushed cardamom seed (must be the seed
inside the pod, not the pod itself)
80ml/generous 3 fl oz virgin olive oil
2 tsp cider vinegar
1 tsp yeastfree tamari

Combine all the ingredients in a screw-top jar and shake well. Store in the fridge and use within 3 weeks.

Sunflower Lime and Ginger Dressing ✓

GLUTENFREE, DAIRYFREE, EGGFREE, YEASTFREE, FC

100 ml/4 fl oz olive oil
$\frac{1}{2}$ tsp grated lime rind
$\frac{1}{2}$ tsp lime juice
2 tsp balsamic vinegar
I tsp tamari
20 roasted sunflower seeds, ground
I tsp grated ginger

Combine all the ingredients in a screw-top jar and shake well. Store in the fridge and use within 3 weeks.

Harissa-style Dressing ✓

serves 4

GLUTENFREE, DAIRYFREE, EGGFREE, YEASTFREE, FC

75ml/3fl oz cold pressed olive oil
6 ripe, deep red tomatoes, chopped
4 garlic cloves, chopped
I tsp cayenne pepper
I tbsp curry powder
2 tbsp lemon juice

Place all the ingredients in of a food processor or blender and blend until smooth. Serve with Roast Vegetable Quinoa Salad or Spicy Lentil Burgers.

Cook's note
Cayenne stimulates the production of hydrochloric acid. If you want to use this recipe but find it too hot, reduce the amount of cayenne pepper to taste.

Thai Green Curry Paste

GLUTENFREE,DAIRYFREE, EGGFREE,YEASTFREE, FC

---

knob of fresh ginger, peeled and finely chopped
3 small pickling onions or ½ small onion
I tsp ground cumin
I tsp ground coriander
2 garlic cloves
6 turns of black pepper mill
grated rind for I lime
juice of ½ lime
handful of chopped coriander (always use stalks as well)

Place all the ingredients in a food processor or blender and blend until smooth. Add a little olive oil if the bowl is very large and the mixture fails to process. Spoon into a glass jar and keep covered in the fridge for up to 5 days.

Use as a topping for grilled fish and chicken, for flavouring sauces and Thai vegetable curries.

Curried Lentil Gravy ✓

serves 4

GLUTENFREE, DAIRYFREE, EGGFREE,YEASTFREE, FC

225g/8oz brown lentils, soaked overnight with kombu strip
570ml/I pt water
2 tsp olive oil
I medium onion, finely chopped
2 garlic cloves, sliced or chopped
small knob of root ginger, peeled and grated
I tsp mixed ground coriander and cumin
I tsp ground turmeric

Drain the soaked lentils and kombu and rinse well. Return the lentils and kombu to the saucepan with fresh water, bring to the boil, drain, rinse and cook in more water until soft, about 30 minutes. Drain the lentils and kombu and reserve any liquid remaining. Chop the kombu.

Heat the oil and fry the onion, garlic and ginger over moderate heat until transparent. Add the coriander and cumin and turmeric and cook for 2 minutes, until the oil and onion mixture is coated with the spices. Add the lentils and kombu and their cooking liquid or 150ml/¼ pint stock and continue cooking for 5 minutes. Purée in a blender or processor and use as a gravy to pour over vegetables, rice, quinoa, buckwheat or millet.

Mayonnaise   ✓

GLUTENFREE, DAIRYFREE, YEASTFREE, FC

---

2 organic egg yolks
2 tbsp cider vinegar
2 tbsp lemon juice
¼ tsp dry mustard
⅛ tsp cayenne pepper (optional)
2 tsp sea salt or to taste
250 ml/8 fl oz olive oil

Place the egg yolks, vinegar, lemon juice, mustard, cayenne pepper, salt and quarter of the oil in a food processor or blender and blend for 30 seconds. Drizzle the remaining oil through the processor funnel with the machine turning and continue to blend until smooth.

Refrigerate in a screw top jar and use within 2 weeks.

Add crushed garlic, curry powder and chopped coriander for curry mayonnaise to serve over chopped vegetables, chicken or fish.

Lemon and Garlic Sauce   ✓

serves 6–8

GLUTENFREE, DAIRYFREE, EGGFREE, YEASTFREE, FC

---

juice of 2 lemons
150 ml/5 fl oz cold pressed olive oil
3 garlic cloves, crushed
4 tbsp chopped parsley,
4 tbsp chopped dill
1 green chilli, finely chopped and deseeded (optional)
2–3 tbsp water

Mix all the ingredients together except the water. Add the water to dilute to taste.

Use to baste grilled vegetables, meats and fish or as a marinade.

Almond Pesto   ✓

serves 4

GLUTENFREE, DAIRYFREE, EGGFREE, YEASTFREE, FC

50g/2oz basil leaves
1 large garlic clove, crushed
50g/2oz blanched almonds
6 tbsp olive oil
sea salt and black pepper
25g/1oz grated hard goat's cheese (stage 1 and 3 only)

Put all the ingredients except the cheese, if using, in a food processor and blend until you have a smooth sauce. Sprinkle the grated cheese over the sauce when combining it with the main ingredients – cooked meat or fish, or vegetables such as courgettes, red peppers or squash. If you are not food combining, toss it through some good quality glutenfree pasta.

Fresh Tomato Sauce with Fennel and Red Pepper

serves 4

GLUTENFREE, DAIRYFREE, EGGFREE, YEAST FREE, FC

900g/2lb tomatoes, skinned and chopped
1 tbsp olive oil
1 large onion, finely chopped
2 garlic cloves, sliced
1 fennel bulb , chopped small
2 red peppers, chopped small
1 tbsp chopped basil
sea salt and black pepper

To skin the tomatoes, pour boiling water over them, leave for 40 seconds and lift them out with a slotted spoon as they will be hot. Slip off the skins off and chop them roughly. If you are a purist, remove the seeds as well.

Heat the oil and sauté the onion and garlic for 3 minutes. Add the chopped fennel and cook for a further 6 minutes until it has softened. Add the red peppers, tomatoes and basil, stir well, cover and simmer gently for 20 minutes. Uncover and continue cooking for another 15 minutes to allow the sauce to reduce and thicken. When cool, process in batches. Taste and add a little sea salt and black pepper if needed.

The flavours will develop if the sauce is left for a few hours or overnight. Freeze any remaining, do not store in the fridge for more than 2 days.

Serve with rice, on vegetables or with glutenfree pasta.

Tomatoes are an acid-forming fruit and therefore are advised for occasional use only. Use fresh, deep red ripe, but firm tomatoes (not orange which may be under-ripe or very acidic or squishy ones which are over-ripe and may be bruised and have mould).

Cook's note

Most tomato sauce recipes have added sugar. By adding fennel and peppers a more balanced, less acid taste is achieved so you don't need to add a sweetener. The fennel, as a member of the dill family, has been used in traditional medicine across the world since ancient times to aid digestion. Dill is a component of baby's gripe water; *dilla* means to lull in Anglo-Saxon.

Avocado Sauce   ✓

serves 4

GLUTENFREE, DAIRYFREE, EGGFREE, YEASTFREE, FC

I large ripe avocado
I tbsp lemon juice
grated rind of $\frac{1}{2}$ lemon
$\frac{1}{2}$ garlic clove, crushed
Sea Vegetable Seasoning
black pepper
150 g/5 oz live plain yoghurt
1 tbsp chopped coriander or parsley

Cut the avocado in half. Remove the stone and peel off the skin, or scrape the flesh out with a spoon. Mash with a fork together with the lemon juice and rind, garlic and seasonings. Add the live yoghurt and chopped herbs to make a pale green creamy sauce.

Serve as a vegetable dip or salad dressing or to accompany salmon, trout or even tinned tuna.

Soups

Sprouted Mung Bean, Celery and Green Bean Soup ✓

serves 4

GLUTENFREE, DAIRYFREE, EGGFREE, YEASTFREE, FC

110g/4oz green beans, tailed
2 tbsp olive oil and ghee, mixed
1 large onion, chopped
4 garlic cloves, chopped
½ head of celery, chopped small
900ml/1½ pts yeastfree vegetable stock
2 tbsp yeastfree tamari
sprouted mung beans, about 1–2 cupfuls
bunch of parsley, chopped

Cut the beans into three-quarter lengths. Heat the oil and ghee in a large pan. Add the onion and garlic and fry gently until transparent. Add the chopped celery and continue cooking for 3 minutes. Add the yeastfree stock, bring to the boil and simmer, covered, for 20 minutes. Add the tamari and mung beans and cook gently for a further 5 minutes until the beans are tender. Stir the chopped parsley through the soup and pour into individual bowls. Alternatively, to speed up digestion, purée the whole soup in a processor or blender.

Chicken Soup ✓

serves 4–6

GLUTENFREE, DAIRYFREE, EGGFREE, YEASTFREE, FC

High food value – easy to absorb nutrition, the favourite medicine of Jewish mothers for coughs and colds.

---

2 medium onions sliced
4 carrots, peeled
½ head of celery, chopped (including green tops)
knob of root ginger, peeled and halved
whole garlic bulb
sprigs of herbs – parsley, rosemary and thyme
1 small/medium organic chicken, the best you can afford
water

The quickest method of making this soup (and all other soups for that matter) is to use a pressure cooker. Make a bed of onions, whole carrots and celery. Add the 2 halves of ginger. Cut off the top of the whole garlic bulb and place both pieces, cut side up, on top of the vegetables; cover with the sprigs of fresh herbs.

Remove chicken giblets and any string or rubber bands from the chicken. Sit the chicken, breast up, on the vegetables. Fill the cooker no more than half full with water and replace the lid securely. From now on follow the instructions for your particular cooker as they all vary. A guide for cooking time at full pressure would be about 8 minutes per lb weight of chicken. If cooking conventionally, cook for one hour in a large covered pan on top of the oven.

Cook's note
When cooked, I do not de-pressurize but leave the lid on to reduce pressure naturally, which also allows the chicken connective tissue to tenderise and the flavour of the stock to intensify. Lift the chicken out and place on a dish. Remove the

ginger pieces and herbs. Now you have four options. (1–3 are suitable for Stage 2.)

1. The liquid stock can be consumed as a consommé with some pieces of vegetables ladled in, with or without some pieces of chicken.
2. You can purée the vegetables with the stock, with or without some chopped chicken, to make a thick soup. Squeeze out the cooked garlic from the cloves and add to the processor.
3. Keep the stock for later (in the fridge or freezer). Carve some chicken and eat with lots of cooked vegetables, adding some steamed broccoli or other green vegetables to boost levels of calcium, folic acid and zinc.

   I do recommend you always store the stocks and water in which you've cooked vegetables and meat as a base for another dish.
4. To cook chicken in vegetable sauce: In a pan slake 2 tbsp corn-flour with 3 tbsp cooled chicken stock. Add 150 ml/5 fl oz more cool stock. Place the pan on the heat to bring the sauce to a simmer. Beating all the time, bring to a boil for about 30 seconds when the stock will be thick and glossy. Add pieces of the vegetables and some diced chicken. Serve with broccoli, courgettes or green beans.

Green Soup   ✓

serves 4

GLUTENFREE, DAIRYFREE, EGGFREE, YEASTFREE, FC

2 tbsp olive oil and ghee, mixed
6 spring onions or 1 leek, chopped
175g/6 oz potatoes, preferably red skinned, cubed
150g/5oz shredded green leaves such as lettuce or spinach
570ml/1 pt vegetable or homemade chicken stock
2 tbsp chopped herbs – watercress, parsley, chervil, dill,
coriander, chives, whatever is available

Heat the olive oil and ghee in a pan and sauté the onions and cubed potatoes for about 4 minutes. Add the shredded green leaves and the stock. Bring to the boil and immediately turn down to a simmer for 8 minute, or until the potatoes are done. Pour the contents into a food processor along with the herbs and whizz until smooth and speckled with herbs.

Mixed Onion Soup   ✓

serves 4

GLUTENFREE, DAIRYFREE, EGGFREE, YEASTFREE, FC

60ml/2½ fl oz olive oil or ghee
450 g/1 lb mixed white, red, Spanish and
English onions finely sliced
4 garlic cloves, finely sliced (not crushed)
900ml/1½ pts yeastfree vegetable stock
2 tbsp yeastfree tamari
1 carrot, peeled and cut into fine rounds

Heat the oil in a large, heavy pan. Add all the onions and swish around with a wooden spatula to coat with oil. Add the garlic and continue cooking and occasionally swishing around until the onions are a light brown, about 15 minutes. Add the vegetable stock and tamari, bring to the boil and cook at a simmer for a further 20 minutes. Take the carrot rounds and cut into fine matchsticks. Ladle the soup into bowls and garnish with carrot.

Cook's note
This recipe introduces two fancy varieties of onion you may not be familiar with. Red and white onions are sweeter than our brown skinned ones and very good eaten raw like Spanish onions. Cooked long and slow till brown like this, you get concentrated sweetness from conversions of carbohydrate to fructose, and an excellent aid to deep sleep.

Celeriac, Parsley and Lemon Soup ✓

serves 4

GLUTENFREE, DAIRYFREE, EGGFREE, YEASTFREE, FC

I tbsp olive oil of ghee
I medium onion, chopped
450g/I lb celeriac, peeled and chopped
½ head of celery, chopped
175g/6oz potato, peeled and chopped
900ml/I ½ pts yeastfree vegetable stock
grated rind of I lemon
4 tbsp mixed chopped parsley, chervil and dill

Heat the oil in a large pan and fry the onion gently until transparent. Add the other vegetables and the stock. Bring to the boil and simmer for 20 minutes until all the vegetables are cooked. Purée the soup in a processor or blender with the lemon rind and herbs until speckled green.

Chickpea and Carrot Soup ✓

serves 4

GLUTENFREE, DAIRYFREE, EGGFREE, YEASTFREE, FC

I tbsp olive oil or ghee
450g/I lb carrots, peeled and sliced
I large onion, chopped
4 garlic cloves, sliced
I tsp ground coriander
I tsp ground cumin
900ml/I ½ pts vegetable stock
415g/15 oz tin chickpeas, drained
I tsp sesame oil
chopped coriander

Heat the oil in a large pan. Add the carrots, onion and garlic and cook gently for 5 minutes, until the onions are transparent. Add the spices and cook for 3 minutes to release their aromatic oils. Add the stock and bring to the boil, stirring constantly. Simmer, covered, for 40 minutes. Add the chickpeas and reheat, stirring well.

Purée in a blender or food processor until smooth. Add the sesame oil and chopped coriander and continue blending until the soup is speckled green.

Onion Soup with Spinach, ✓ Spring Onions and Ginger

serves 4

GLUTENFREE, DAIRYFREE, EGGFREE, YEASTFREE, FC

---

2 tbsp olive oil
250g/9 oz onions, finely sliced
4 garlic cloves, finely sliced (not crushed)
900ml/1 ½ pts vegetable stock
1 tsp grated root ginger
2tbsp frozen spinach (or small bunch of chopped fresh)
2 spring onions, finely chopped

Heat the oil in a large, heavy pan. Add the sliced onions and swish around with a wooden spatula to coat with oil. Add the garlic and continue cooking over moderate heat, swishing until the onions have turned brown about 20 minutes. Add the vegetable stock and grated ginger, bring to the boil, and cook at a simmer for a further 15 minutes. Add the spinach, stir well and cook for 5 minutes. Ladle the soup into bowls and garnish with chopped spring onion.

Two Pea Mint, Coriander and Lemon Soup

serves 4–6

GLUTENFREE, DAIRYFREE, EGGFREE, YEASTFREE

110g/4oz potato, peeled and diced
1 medium onion, sliced
1.1 1/2 pts vegetable or chicken stock
knob of fresh ginger, peeled and grated
$\frac{1}{2}$ tsp ground coriander
2 tsp ground cumin
4 tbsp chopped coriander
$\frac{1}{2}$ tsp cayenne pepper (optional)
350g/12oz fresh or frozen peas
pinch of sea salt
1 tbsp lemon juice
grated rind of 1 lemon
10 mange touts, for garnish
4 sprigs of mint

Combine the first six ingredients in a pan and bring to the boil. Cover and simmer for 30 minutes. Add the chopped coriander, cayenne, peas, sea salt, lemon juice and rind and return to the boil. Reduce the heat and simmer for several minutes until the peas are tender.

Purée the soup in a processor or blender until smooth. Return to the pan, reheat, adding the mange touts, and cook for 2 minutes. Serve in bowls, garnished with little sprigs of mint.

Cook's note
This can be adapted for use at Stage 2 by omitting the potato.

Spinach, Calabrese and Tarragon Soup

serves 4

GLUTENFREE, DAIRYFREE, EGGFREE, YEASTFREE, FATFREE, FC

110g/4oz potato, chopped small
700ml/1¼ pts yeastfree stock
450g/1 lb calabrese broccoli, divided into
small florets, plus stalk slices
225g/8 oz spinach, washed
1 tsp green peppercorns, ground (optional)
1 tbsp yeastfree tamari
2 tsp chopped tarragon or 1 tsp dried tarragon
2 tbsp spring onions, finely chopped
1 dsp Sea Vegetable Seasoning
1 tsp finely chopped chives

Put the potato and stock into a pan and simmer for 5 minutes. Add the calabrese and spinach, bring to the boil and simmer for a further 10 minutes.

Purée in a food processor or blender. Return the soup to the pan and add the crushed peppercorns, if using, tamari, tarragon, spring onions and sea vegetable seasoning. Serve garnished with chives.

Hurdy Gurdy Soup (Basic Vegetable Soup)✓

serves 4

GLUTENFREE, DAIRYFREE, EGGFREE, YEASTFREE, FC

1.4kg/3lb mixed vegetables, whatever you have in the fridge
2 tbsp olive oil
1.1 1/2 pts yeastfree vegetable stock
2 tbsp fresh or 1 tbsp dried mixed herbs
1 tbsp yeastfree tamari
black pepper

This is a good, basic vegetable soup. Peel and dice the root vegetables to roughly the same size. Trim any green vegetables of their outer leaves and wash thoroughly under cold water. Cut into small florets, sprigs or slices. Leave to drain.

Heat the oil in a large pan. Add the root vegetables and sauté for 5 minutes until transparent. Add the stock, bring to the boil and simmer for 10 minutes. Add the green vegetables and herbs and continue cooking for another 10 minutes or until the greens are tender. Season to taste with the tamari and black pepper.

Serve straight away as is or put through a food processor or blender in batches to make a creamier soup. Serve with Savoury Vegetable Pancakes (Stages 1 and 3 only).

Sweet Pea and Coconut Soup

serves 4

GLUTENFREE, DAIRYFREE, EGGFREE, YEASTFREE, FC

---

1 tbsp olive oil or ghee
110 g/4oz fresh or frozen peas
110 g/4oz fresh or frozen green beans
125g/4oz fresh or frozen broad beans
6 spring onions, finely chopped
1/2 tsp ground coriander
pinch of grated nutmeg
570ml/1 pt yeastfree vegetable stock
275ml/10 fl oz coconut milk
6 lettuce leaves

Heat the oil in a large pan, add all the vegetables and cook quickly for 3 minutes without browning , stirring constantly. Add the coriander and a pinch of nutmeg. Cook for another 2 minutes. Add the stock, coconut milk and the lettuce leaves and simmer for 10 minutes until all the vegetables are soft.

Purée the soup in a processor or blender until smooth. Return to the pan and reheat gently before serving.

Salads

Roast Vegetable Quinoa Salad ✓

serves 4

GLUTENFREE, DAIRYFREE, EGGFREE, YEASTFREE, FC

I small bulb of fennel, quartered
450g/1lb ripe, deep red tomatoes
I small aubergine, chopped
3 courgettes, chopped
2 red peppers, cubed
I Spanish onion, quartered
8 garlic cloves, unpeeled and halved
bunch of basil leaves
4 tbsp olive oil
black pepper
275g/10oz quinoa
I tbsp cold pressed olive oil
selection of mixed green salad leaves
Harissa-style Dressing

Preheat the oven to 240C, 475F. Gas Mark 9.

Separate the fennel leaves. Place all the vegetables and garlic evenly in a roasting tin. Tear up half the bunch of basil and scatter over the vegetables. Drizzle over the olive oil and turn over the vegetables to coat. Roast for 35–45 minutes (depending on your oven), until the vegetables are beginning to brown. (Turn once while cooking.) Remove the vegetables to a bowl and leave to cool.

While the vegetables are roasting, cook the quinoa. Rinse the grains under cold running water for several minutes. Cover the quinoa with water in a medium pan, bring to the boil and simmer for 20–25 minutes until tender. Drain well. Pour the cold pressed olive oil into the warm pan and return the quinoa to it, stirring through with a wooden spoon. Turn on to a large serving plate and leave to cool.

To serve, arrange the roasted vegetables over the quinoa and top with the salad leaves. Finally, dress the leaves with some Harissa-style dressing or an alternative of your choice.

Cook's note
For a Stage 1 or Stage 3 treat dot with a little goat's cheese.

Celeriac, Carrot and Mayonnaise Salad

serves 4

GLUTENFREE, DAIRYFREE, YEASTFREE, FC

350g/12oz celeriac or daikon, peeled and grated
3 carrots, scrubbed and grated
1 parsnip, peeled and grated
juice and grated rind of 1 lime
3 tbsp Mayonnaise (see page 132)
1 tbsp grain mustard
25g/1oz chopped almonds
2 tbsp chopped parsley
2 tbsp finely chopped chives

Mix the grated roots with the lime juice and rind. Add the remaining ingredients and mix well together.

Cook's note
Stage 2 – omit parsnip

Avocado and Green Pea ✓
Guacamole Dip

serves 4

GLUTENFREE, DAIRYFREE (IF USING GOAT'S YOGHURT),
EGGFREE, YEASTFREE, FC

225g/8oz frozen peas, thawed
1 large avocado, peeled and stoned
3 garlic cloves
1 tsp Sea Vegetable Seasoning
4 tbsp lime juice
grated rind of 1 lime
4 tbsp goat's yoghurt
4 tbsp finely copped coriander
1 tbsp chopped fine mint

Mash the peas with the avocado. Peel the garlic, slice finely and then chop very finely. Add to the avocado with the sea vegetable seasoning, lime juice and grated rind. Mix well. Fold in the yoghurt – just sufficient to loosen the guacamole to a soft, dropping consistency. Add the chopped coriander and mint.

Serve with vegetable sticks in a lunch box, as a first course or as part of a curry meal.

Grated Carrot with Sesame Seeds ✓

serves 1

GLUTENFREE, DAIRYFREE, EGGFREE, YEASTFREE, FC

---

2 carrots, scrubbed and grated
1 dsp chives
2 tsp sesame seeds
1 tsp sesame oil
1 dsp olive oil

Put the carrots in a bowl and scissor over the chives. Add the sesame seeds and oils, and mix well. Serve with any dish on the diet.

Celery, Cucumber and Red Onion Salsa ✓

serves 4

GLUTENFREE, DAIRYFREE, EGGFREE, YEASTFREE, FC

1/3 cucumber, peeled and roughly chopped
3 small celery sticks, roughly chopped
1/4 red onion, roughly chopped

Place all the ingredients in a food processor or blender and process until finely chopped.

Serve with Thai Fishcakes, Grilled Chicken Pieces or Mixed Vegetable Curry.

Avocado, Tomato, Cucumber, ✓ Basil and Alfalfa Salad

serves 1

GLUTENFREE, DAIRYFREE, EGGFREE, YEASTFREE, FC

1/2 ripe avocado, peeled and sliced
I medium ripe, deep red tomato, sliced
6 slices cucumber, peeled
basil leaves
alfalfa sprouts
Herb Dressing

Arrange the slices of avocado, tomato and cucumber on a plate and decorate with basil leaves and alfalfa sprouts. Drizzle over some Herb Dressing and serve.

Winter Coleslaw with Sea Vegetables, ✓ Mustard and Lemon

serves 4

GLUTENFREE, DAIRYFREE, EGGFREE, YEASTFREE, FC

225g/8oz carrots, and grated
110g/4oz parsnip, peeled and grated
110g/4oz swede, peeled and grated
110g/4oz red or white cabbage, finely sliced
110g/4oz celery or daikon, finely chopped
8 spring onions or ½ mild salad onion, finely sliced
2 tbsp yeastfree tamari
1 tbsp best olive oil
1 tsp wholegrain mustard
1 tsp cider vinegar
grated rind of 1 lemon
1 dsp linseeds
1 tbsp Sea Vegetable Seasoning
2 tbsp sunflower seeds
1 tbsp pumpkin seeds
1 tbsp almonds

Discard outer leaves of red cabbage before slicing. Mix all the prepared vegetables together in a large bowl. Blend the tamari, oil, mustard, cider vinegar and lemon rind together in another bowl or jam jar with lid. Process the linseeds in a coffee grinder until finely ground and add to the dressing. Stir in the sea vegetable seasoning. Add the sunflower and pumpkin seeds and almonds to the vegetables. Pour the dressing over the vegetables and stir through all the ingredients.

Store in a covered bowl in the fridge.

Cook's note

This salad is excellent for lunch boxes and picnics. It will keep for 2 days in the fridge, so it makes sense to make a large quantity like this at one time.

The seeds and almonds make up a whole protein salad.

Without breaking the food combining code you could add chicken or eggs for a main course.

Italian Vegetable Salad   ✓

serves 4

GLUTENFREE, DAIRYFREE, EGGFREE, YEASTFREE, FC

---

2 medium red peppers
2 medium aubergines
1 tbsp olive oil
1 onion, finely chopped
1 carrot, peeled and sliced
1 celery stick, sliced
3 courgettes, sliced
8 (about 900g/2lb) medium ripe,
deep red tomatoes, chopped
3 tbsp water
1 tbsp cider vinegar
bunch of basil leaves

Heat the grill to its highest setting and grill the skin of the red peppers and aubergines until they are brown all over. Place in a bowl and cover until cool. Skin the peppers and chop into squares. Scoop out the flesh from the aubergine skins and chop roughly.

Heat the oil in a pan. Add the onion and fry for 5 minutes until transparent. Add the carrot, celery, courgettes and peppers and continue to fry until soft. Add the aubergine and chopped tomatoes with the water and simmer for 30 minutes until thick. Cool. Add the cider vinegar. Store in the fridge. Garnish with basil leaves when serving.

Preferably prepare this salad the day before eating to allow the flavours to mature. Serve with a mixed green salad with Harissa-style Dressing, rice or other grain.

Quinoa Salad Tabbouleh-style ✓

serves 4

GLUTENFREE, DAIRYFREE, EGGFREE, YEASTFREE, FC

I cup (measuring or tea cup) quinoa
2½ cups (as above) water
50g/2oz parsley, chopped
8 spring onions, chopped
4 tbsp lemon juice
450g/Ilb ripe, cherry tomatoes, chopped
bunch of mint, destalked and chopped
¼ cucumber, skinned and diced
2 tbsp extra virgin olive oil
sea salt and black pepper

Cook the quinoa gently in the water until transparent, about 25 minutes. Remove from the heat and leave for 10–15 minutes to fluff up. When cool add the other ingredients and season with salt and pepper.

Serve with mixed salad or another Middle Eastern type recipe such as Butterbean, Aubergine and Celeriac Purée.

Mediterranean Onion Salad   ✓

serves 4

GLUTENFREE, DAIRYFREE, EGGFREE, YEASTFREE, FC

---

4 tbsp olive oil and ghee, mixed
2 carrots, finely chopped
900g/2lb small pickling onions, peeled
250ml/8 fl oz vegetable stock
4 tbsp cider vinegar
6 ripe, deep red tomatoes, roughly chopped
2 bay leaves
bunch of basil leaves
black pepper

Heat the oil gently in a large pan. Add the carrots and simmer gently for 5 minutes, stirring frequently. Add the onions, stock, cider vinegar, chopped tomatoes and bay leaves. Bring to the boil and simmer, covered, for an hour, until the onions are tender and the sauce is thick. Cool, store in the fridge and use the next day. Garnish with basil leaves and season with black pepper before serving with rice or another grain. Can be served cold as a salad or hot as a sauce.

Cook's note
The bay leaves are left in the salad to enhance the flavour but are not meant to be eaten.

Vegetables

Baked Spanish Onions with Goat's Cheese ✓

serves 4

GLUTENFREE, DAIRYFREE, YEASTFREE, FC

---

4 large Spanish onions, unpeeled
75g/3oz soft goat's cheese
1 organic or free range egg
3 tbsp chopped parsley
¼ tsp mixed dried herbs – thyme and rosemary
2 tbsp extra virgin olive oil

Preheat the oven to 200°C/400°F/Gas Mark 6.

Simmer the onions whole and unpeeled in water for 10 minutes. Drain in a colander and run cold water over them to cool. Carefully peel away the outer skin and then detach the central core to allow for stuffing. Place the onions upright on a baking tray. Finely chop the onion from the central core.

In a bowl, mix the goat's cheese with the egg, herbs and the finely chopped onion and fill the whole onions with the mixture. Brush the onions with the oil, drizzling a little over the stuffing. Bake for 45 minutes. They are delicious either hot or cold.

Serve with a risotto (stages 1 and 3 only), some green vegetables such as broccoli or cabbage, roast lamb, chicken or game.

Asparagus with Tarragon and Lemon ✓

serves 6

GLUTENFREE, DAIRYFREE, EGGFREE, YEASTFREE

---

900 g/2 lb asparagus spears, trimmed
6 sprigs of tarragon, washed
3 lemons, halved
cold pressed olive oil

Bring a large frying pan of water to the boil. Add the asparagus and tarragon sprigs, cover and cook for 5 minutes. refresh the asparagus under cold water and pat dry with a clean tea-towel or kitchen paper. Serve cold with ½ lemon per person and drizzled with cold pressed olive oil. This goes well with slices of avocado, tomato and goat's cheese or grilled chicken or fish.

Potato and Sesame Cakes

makes 6–8 cakes

GLUTENFREE, DAIRYFREE, YEASTFREE

450g/1lb even sized waxy potatoes, peeled and left whole
1 organic or free range egg, beaten
1 tbsp gram (chickpea) flour
1 tbsp sesame seeds
4 spring onions, chopped
1 tbsp chopped parsley
sea salt and black pepper
2 tbsp olive oil and ghee mixed

If the potatoes are uneven in size, cut them to match but keep them as large as possible. Boil the potatoes for 7 minutes, drain and cool. When they are cool enough to handle, either grate them on the coarse side of a cheese grater or push through the grating disc of a food processor. Place in a mixing bowl. Add the beaten egg, flour, sesame seeds, chopped spring onions, parsley and seasoning, and mix well.

With clean hands, squidge 6-8 portions of the mixture together to form cakes. If possible, leave them in the fridge for 10 minutes to firm up slightly. Heat the oil mixture gently in a heavy frying pan and cook 2–3 cakes at a time for 4-5 minutes on each side. Drain on kitchen paper as they are cooked.

Serve with green vegetables or Grated Carrot with Sesame Seeds or a vegetable stir-fry. Alternatively, as this recipe breaks the food combining rules you could serve with some chicken, fish or lentil stew.

Big Root Chips ✓

serves 4

GLUTENFREE, DAIRYFREE, EGGFREE, YEASTFREE, FC

---

4 tbsp olive oil
selection of root vegetables, such as 2 parsnips,
$\frac{1}{2}$ celeriac, 6 carrots, small swede
1 garlic bulb, unpeeled
sprigs of rosemary

Preheat the oven to 200°C/400°F/Gas Mark 6.

Pour the oil on to a thick baking tray and heat in the oven.

Scrub or peel the roots and cut into thick matchsticks ¾ in/1.5 cm thick. Slice the unpeeled garlic into thick rounds.

Carefully take the baking tray out of the oven and arrange layers of roots and garlic evenly over the pan surface. Tuck sprigs of rosemary under the chips. Roast for 30 minutes, turning once until the chips begin to caramelise around the edges. Discard the rosemary.

Serve immediately with a herby salad of rocket, cos lettuce, tarragon and wilted raddiccio.

Cook's note
At stages 1 and 3 you can dotted with goat's cheese and black olives.

Baked Potatoes Stuffed with ✓ Spring Onions, Celery and Broccoli

serves 2

GLUTENFREE, DAIRYFREE, EGGFREE, YEASTFREE, FC

---

2 baking potatoes
2 celery sticks, chopped
4 broccoli florets
2 spring onions, chopped
Sea Vegetable Seasoning

Bake the potatoes by your favourite method. While they are cooking, boil the celery and broccoli for 5 minutes in a little water and drain. When the potatoes are cooked, split them open and stuff the spring onions, celery and broccoli into the cavity and sprinkle on some sea vegetable seasoning.

Serve immediately with salad or Mange-tout, Asparagus and Spring Onion Stir-fry.

Colcannon ✓

serves 4

GLUTENFREE, DAIRYFREE, EGGFREE, YEASTFREE, FC

---

5 fl oz/150 mls water
450g/1 lb green cabbage, finely shredded
700g/1 ½ lb hot mashed potato
2 tbsp chopped spring onion
2 tbsp olive oil

Put some water in a pan and bring to the boil. Add the cabbage and cook fast for 3–4 minutes, stirring constantly. Drain and add to the mashed potato with all the other ingredients. Beat together and serve.

Turnip Mash with Nutmeg ✓

serves 4

GLUTENFREE, DAIRYFREE, EGGFREE, YEASTFREE, FC

---

4 medium turnips, peeled and quartered
knob of butter or 1 tsp olive oil
a little sea salt and black pepper
freshly grated nutmeg

Steam the turnips until soft, about 20 minutes. Mash well until smooth. Turn them into a warm dish and stir in the butter or olive oil, sea salt and black pepper. Add lots of grated nutmeg and serve.

Cauliflower with Coriander and ✓ Sunflower Seeds

serves 4

GLUTENFREE, DAIRYFREE, EGGFREE, YEASTFREE, FC

---

1 large cauliflower
2 tbsp sunflower seeds
1 tsp coriander seeds
2 tbsp olive oil
1 large onion, chopped
2 garlic cloves, crushed
sea salt and black pepper

Separate the cauliflower into small florets plus the stalks. Rinse well. Heat a heavy frying pan and dry roast the sunflower and coriander seeds for about 3 minutes, shaking the pan frequently. When cool, grind both seeds in a coffee grinder or food processor.

Heat the oil in the same pan and fry off the onion until translucent. Turn up the heat and add the cauliflower, sautéing with the onion for about 5 minutes. Stir in the crushed garlic and cook for another minute. Add the crushed seeds and move the mixture around until the cauliflower and onion are speckled.

Cook's note

Serve with fish or chicken which will veer slightly off the food combining route because of the sunflower seeds with the cauliflower. At Stage 2, leave them out or just serve another vegetable.

Broccoli and Shitake Mushroom Stir-fry

serves 4

GLUTENFREE, DAIRYFREE, EGGFREE, YEASTFREE, FC

---

2 tbsp olive oil
8 spring onions, chopped
4 garlic cloves, sliced
450g/1lb broccoli, divided into small florets
20 g/1½ oz dried shitake mushrooms
(soaked for 20 minutes in warm water)
2 tbsp yeastfree tamari

Heat the wok. Add the oil and cook the spring onions until wilted. Stir in the garlic and cook for 1 minute. Stir in the broccoli and cook for 2 minutes. Add the shitake mushrooms and the soaking liquid. Toss this mixture around in the wok for about 3 minutes until the broccoli is crunchy but not raw. Swirl through the tamari. Turn up the heat to high for a few seconds at the end of cooking.

Nice with grilled chicken as a quick supper.

Cook's note

Dried shitake mushrooms have immune-system-building properties and are the only mushrooms suitable for the *Beat Candida Diet*.

Carrot, Broccoli and Parsnip Korma

serves 4

GLUTENFREE, DAIRYFREE, EGGFREE, YEASTFREE, FC

275g/10oz carrots, sliced
275g/10oz parsnips, peeled
4 tbsp olive oil
1 large onion, chopped
4 garlic cloves, finely chopped
1 tbsp ground cumin
1 dsp ground coriander
1 dsp turmeric
small knob of fresh ginger, peeled and grated
275 ml/10 fl oz live plain yoghurt
50g/2oz ground almonds
275ml/10floz vegetable stock
350g/12oz broccoli, divided into florets
small bunch of coriander, chopped

Cut the carrots and parsnips to a similar size.

Heat the oil in a large saucepan. Add the onion and fry until golden brown. Add the garlic and shortly afterwards, the spices and ginger. Keep stirring and cooking until the spices begin to form a sticky paste. Take the pan off the heat and stir in the yoghurt, scraping around the pan to pick up the spices and blend into a sauce. Add the almonds and stir again. Return to the heat and bring very slowly up to a simmer. Stir in the stock.

Add the carrots and parsnips, stirring well. Cover the pan and cook gently for 15 minutes. Add the broccoli and cook for 10 minutes. Just before serving, add the chopped coriander and cook for 3 more minutes. Ideal with a salad or another vegetable.

Cooks note

For a non-food combining alternative, serve with brown rice. Alternatively, add some cooked chicken with the coriander just before serving.

Mange-tout, Asparagus and Spring Onion Stir fry

serves 4

GLUTENFREE, DAIRYFREE, EGGFREE, YEASTFREE, FC

---

1 tbsp olive oil or ghee
225g/8oz baby asparagus
12 spring onions, finely chopped
225g/8oz mange touts, trimmed
1 tbsp yeastfree tamari
2 tbsp water
1 tsp Sea Vegetable Seasoning
1 tsp sesame oil

Heat the wok and add the oil. Add the asparagus and stir-fry for 4 minutes, tossing constantly. Add the spring onions and 1 minute later add the mange touts. Stir-fry for about 3 minutes until the asparagus has begun to soften but is still crunchy. Add the remaining ingredients and stir-fry for 3 minutes.

Serve with grilled chicken or fish.

Steamed Broccoli and Leeks   ✓

serves 2

GLUTENFREE, DAIRYFREE, EGGFREE, YEASTFREE, FC

---

250 g/9 oz broccoli florets
175 g/6 oz leeks, halved and finely sliced
water

Steam the broccoli and leeks for 4–5 minutes until both vegetables are tender. Arrange the leeks on a serving plate, surrounded by broccoli, topped with Almond Pesto.

Grilled Fennel and Goat's Cheese   ✓

serves 4

GLUTENFREE, DAIRYFREE, EGGFREE, YEASTFREE, FC

---

4 medium fennel bulbs
2 tbsp olive oil
110g/4oz soft goat's cheese

Trim the fennel bulbs, removing the tough outer layer and the green fronds. Keep the outer layer for tomorrow's soup and the fronds for garnish. Halve the bulbs lengthwise. Place in a steamer and cook for 10 minutes. Drain.

Heat the grill to its highest setting. Arrange the fennel on the grill rack, brush with olive oil and grill for 5 minutes until the bulbs begin to brown. Divide the goat's cheese into eight and spread over the hot fennel halves. The heat will be sufficient to melt the cheese.

Serve with Brown Rice with Whole Garlic and Lemon (stages 1 and 3 only), mixed with a green vegetable such as broccoli, green beans or courgettes.

Asparagus and Courgette Risotto   ✓

serves 4

GLUTENFREE, DAIRYFREE, EGGFREE, YEASTFREE, FC

450g/1lb asparagus, trimmed
225g/8oz courgettes, sliced
2tbsp olive oil
1 medium onion, finely chopped
2 garlic cloves, crushed
350g/12oz brown short-grain rice
1.1 1/2 pts vegetable stock
2 tbsp chopped herbs – mint, parsley, chives

Cut the asparagus into short lengths. Bring a pan of water to the boil and cook the asparagus pieces and courgettes for 5 minutes. Drain and reserve liquid . Heat the oil in a pan. Add the onion and garlic and fry for 3–5 minutes, until softened. Add the rice and stir well until coated with oil. Add the stock and asparagus water gradually over the next 20 minutes until the rice becomes tender and creamy. Stir in the herbs and vegetables, and stir to reheat. Serve with baked onions, Big Root Chips (stages 1 and 3 only) or more green vegetables.

Spicy Aubergine and Potato Crust   ✓

serves 4

GLUTENFREE, DAIRYFREE, EGGFREE, YEASTFREE, FC

700g/1½ lb potatoes, peeled and cubed
knob of butter or 1 tsp olive oil
2–3 aubergines (about 1 kg/2¼ lb)
1 tsp olive oil
2 medium onions, sliced
3 garlic cloves, finely sliced
1 tbsp garam masala
1 dsp turmeric
1 tsp ground cumin
1 tsp ground coriander
225g/8oz chopped tomatoes
125 ml/4 fl oz vegetable or chicken stock
2 tbsp chopped parsley
2 spring onion, finely chopped
Preheat the grill to its highest setting.

Preheat oven to 200°C/400°F/Gas Mark 6. Boil the potatoes in a minimum of water until tender, about 10 minutes. Drain and mash, then beat in the butter or oil. Cover and set aside. Grill the whole aubergines, turning frequently until the skin blisters and blackens. Remove from the grill and leave to cool.

Heat the oil in a pan. Add the onions and garlic and sautée until translucent. Add the garam masala, turmeric, cumin and coriander and cook for 2–3 minutes to blend the spice flavours together.

Split the aubergines, scoop out the soft pulp and add to the spiced onions and garlic. Stir well, then add the tomatoes and stock. Cook for a further 20 minutes. Add the chopped parsley and spoon this mixture into an ovenproof dish. Beat the chopped spring onions into the mashed potato and layer on top of the aubergine mixture, forking up the potato in peaks.

Put into the oven and cook for 25 minutes. Serve with some green vegetables.

Stir fried Cabbage with Lime and Coconut

serves 4

GLUTENFREE, DAIRYFREE, EGGFREE, YEASTFREE, FC

450g/1 lb spring greens or pointed cabbage
2 tbsp olive oil or ghee
2 tsp Thai Green Curry Paste or
ready-made paste
150ml/5 fl oz coconut milk
grated rind and juice of 1 lime
black pepper

Shred the greens or cabbage finely. Heat the wok, add the oil and stir fry the cabbage for 3–4 minutes until wilted. Mix together the Thai paste, coconut milk, grated lime and 1 tbsp of lime juice, pour into the wok and bring to the boil. Cook for 3–4 minutes until the greens are tender.

Serve with grilled fish or chicken.

Mixed Vegetable Curry   ✓

serves 6

GLUTENFREE, DAIRYFREE, EGGFREE, YEASTFREE, FC

---

2 large onions, chopped
4 garlic cloves
2 tbsp vegetable stock
2 tbsp olive oil
1 tbsp ground coriander
2 tsp cumin seeds
1 tbsp curry powder
1/2 tsp chilli powder (optional)
110 g/4 oz baby sweetcorn
175 g/6 oz courgettes, sliced
small savoy cabbage, cut into chunks
2 red peppers, chopped small
6 ripe, deep red tomatoes
250 ml/8fl oz hot yeastfree vegetable stock
2 tbsp chopped coriander

Blend the onions, garlic and stock in a food processor or blender and whizz to a smooth paste.

Heat the oil in a heavy pan and fry the spices for about 2 minutes. Add the onion mixture, stir well and cook for 3 minutes. Add the vegetables and sauté for 5 minutes. Pour on the hot stock, stirring to blend the flavours together. Simmer for 20 minutes. Garnish with chopped coriander before serving with rice or other grain.

This recipe will develop its flavours well if left to be eaten until the following day.

It freezes well for 3 weeks.

Cabbage, Almond and Beansprout Parcels ✓

serves 4

GLUTENFREE, DAIRYFREE, EGGFREE, YEASTFREE, FC

---

8 savoy cabbage leaves or chinese leaves
2 carrots, peeled and finely sliced
50g/2oz sprouted almonds (soaked in water for
12 hours then drained)
110g/4oz organic beansprouts
8 spring onions, finely chopped
2 garlic cloves, grated
knob of ginger, grated
1 tsp yeastfree tamari
2 tsp Sea Vegetable Seasoning
1 tbsp sunflower oil

Preheat the oven to 180°C/350°F/Gas Mark 4.

Blanch the cabbage or chinese leaves in boiling water for 2 minutes until wilted. Plunge into cold water to cool. Drain and pat dry with a clean tea-towel.

Mix all the other ingredients together in a bowl. Take about an eighth of the mixture and place in the centre of a cabbage leaf, then fold up envelope-style into a parcel. Do the same with the other seven leaves. Arrange on a baking tray and cook for 20–25 minutes.

Serve with meat or fish, or add strips of cooked chicken to the parcels.

Cook's note
Supermarket Chinese beansprouts with long thin sprouts have been sprayed with chemicals to kill bacteria – short organic beansprouts sold in healthfood shops are chemical-free.

Seeds, pulses and grains

Cooking Rice

serves 2

GLUTENFREE, DAIRYFREE, EGGFREE, YEASTFREE, FC

Three simple and foolproof ways of cooking rice can be adapted to suit your digestion of grains.

Basic Method
1 cup (measuring or tea cup) brown rice
3 cups (as above) water
1 tsp cold pressed olive oil

Wash the rice thoroughly in a sieve under cold running water. Place in a pan with the water and cook gently, covered, for 35–40 minutes. Rinse with boiling water. Return to the pan, stir in the olive oil and mix to coat.

Method for Better Digestion ✓
1 cup (measuring cup or tea cup) brown rice
5 cups (as above) water
1 tsp cold pressed olive oil

Soak the rice for 10 minutes to 2 hours in cold water. Rinse well. Place in a pan with the water and cook for 30 minutes. Rinse with boiling water. Return to the pan, stir in the olive oil and mix to coat.

Maximum Digestion   ✓

Cook one cup of pre-soaked (as above) rice in a pressure
cooker according the manufacturer's instructions.

With the rice you could also cook some vegetables to make
yourself a quick nutritious meal.

Cooking Quinoa   ✓

serves 2

GLUTENFREE, DAIRYFREE, EGGFREE, YEASTFREE, FC

---

1 cup (measuring or tea cup) quinoa
2½–3 cups (as above) water
1 tsp cold pressed olive oil

Rinse the quinoa well under cold running water, discarding
any grit. Place in a pan with the water and simmer covered, for
25-30 minutes until soft. Take off the heat and leave to fluff up
for 10-15 minutes. Stir in the olive oil and mix to coat.

For a quick meal put some chopped up vegetables on top of
the quinoa so they cook in the steam.

Brown Rice with Whole Garlic   ✓
and Lemon

serves 4

GLUTENFREE, DAIRYFREE, EGGFREE, YEASTFREE, FC

---

4 garlic cloves, unpeeled
2 tbsp olive oil
350g/12oz brown rice, rinsed
1 l/1¾ pts water
1 dsp cold pressed olive oil
juice of 1 lemon
grated rind of 1 lemon
2 tbsp chopped parsley

Preheat the oven to 230C, 450F, Gas Mark 8.

Arrange the whole garlic cloves on a baking tray, brush the ordinary with olive oil and place in the oven. Reduce the heat to 200°C/400°F/Gas Mark 6 and roast for 25 minutes.

While the garlic is roasting, cook the rinsed rice in the water, covered, for about 45 minutes, until the rice is well done. Drain and rinse with boiling water. Rinse the pan and return the rice to it. Add the cold pressed olive oil, lemon juice and rind, and stir quickly through the rice until well mixed. Turn off the heat, stir through the parsley. Cut the tops off the garlic and squeeze out the cooked cloves into the rice. Serve.

Cook's note

This is simple and helpful recipe. There is good acid/alkaline balance between the acid, carbohydrate rice and alkaline lemon plus anti-fungal, detoxing garlic, blood purifying parsley and full strength oleic acid from the cold pressed olive oil.

Tamari Seeds ✓

GLUTENFREE, DAIRYFREE, EGGFREE, YEASTFREE
(IF USING YEASTFREE TAMARI), FC

200 g/7 oz pumpkin seeds
200 g/7 oz sunflower seeds
2 tbsp yeastfree Tamari

Preheat the oven to 150°C/300°F/Gas Mark 2.

Mix the two seeds together on a large baking tray and roast for 20 minutes.

Sprinkle over the tamari and turn over the seeds to coat with the sauce. Return to the oven for 5 minutes. Remove from the oven and leave to cool before storing in a screw-top glass jar.

Smaller quantities may be made in a frying pan, stirring for 5 minutes and adding the tamari at the end.

Red Peppers Stuffed with Rice and Almonds

serves 4

GLUTENFREE, DAIRYFREE, EGGFREE, YEASTFREE

---

5 red peppers
2 tbsp olive oil
2 courgettes, diced
1 large onion, finely chopped
2 garlic cloves, chopped
185 g/6$\frac{1}{2}$ oz brown rice, rinsed
400ml/15 fl oz hot yeastfree vegetable stock
2 tbsp chopped basil
25g/1oz ground almonds
black pepper
50g/2oz soft goat's cheese

Preheat the oven to 190C, 375F, Gas Mark 5.

Deseed and chop up one of the peppers – the least cylindrical one. Slice off the tops of the other peppers and reserve. Carefully pull out seeds and fibrous parts from each pepper and discard. Heat half the olive oil in a pan and fry the chopped pepper and courgettes until soft.

Heat the remaining olive oil in a large pan and fry the onion and garlic until translucent. Add the rinsed rice and stir-fry for 3 minutes. Pour over the stock and simmer, stirring, as if making a risotto, until the rice has absorbed all the liquid. Stir in the pepper and courgette mixture. Add the basil to the pan with the ground almonds and several grinds of black pepper. Mix well.

Place the peppers upright in a baking tray and fill with the rice mixture. Dot with goat's cheese and top with the stalk rings. Bake for 25 minutes. Serve with green salad.

Millet with Courgettes, ✓
Green Beans and Thyme

serves 4

GLUTENFREE, DAIRYFREE, EGGFREE, YEATFREE, FC

I tbsp olive oil
175 g/6 oz millet
I bunch of spring onions, chopped
I medium red pepper, chopped
175 g/6 oz courgettes, thickly sliced
110 g/4 oz green beans
4 ripe, deep red tomatoes, chopped
570 ml/1 pt vegetable stock
2 tsp chopped thyme
grated rind of I large lemon
I tbsp yeastfree tamari
black pepper

Heat the oil in a large pan and lightly toast the millet until it begins to brown. Add the spring onions, red pepper, courgettes, green beans and tomatoes and cook for 7 minutes. Stir in the stock, thyme and lemon rind. Bring to the boil, cover and simmer gently for 20 minutes. Add the yeastfree tamari and several grinds of black pepper.

Cook's note
All one-pot cooking recipes develop their correct flavours after cooking as the mixture of ingredients blend together. For the best results and balance of tastes leave soups, stews and casseroles to eat the day after cooking. In between store in the fridge.

Rice Noodles with Coconut and Almond Cream

serves 4

GLUTENFREE, DAIRYFREE, EGGFREE, YEASTFREE, FC

225g/8oz rice noodles
25g/1oz creamed coconut from block
150ml/5 fl oz boiling water
1 tbsp yeastfree tamari
1 tsp sesame oil
50g/2oz ground almonds
1 tbsp olive oil
8 spring onions, chopped
1 carrot, cut into matchsticks
1 red pepper, thinly sliced
175 g/6 oz leeks, trimmed, halved and finely sliced
½ cucumber, chopped
8 sprigs of coriander, chopped

Place the noodles in a large bowl and just cover them with boiling water. Leave to soak for 10 minutes. Stir with a fork, drain then rinse under cold water. Rinse again and leave to drain.

Mix the creamed coconut with the boiling water in a small pan until dissolved. Stir in the tamari, sesame oil and ground almonds. Heat gently for 4 minutes, then set aside. Heat the wok. Add the oil, then the spring onions, carrot and red pepper and stir fry for 3 minutes. Add the leeks and cook until transparent. Remove from the heat and add the noodles and cucumber. Pour the dressing over the salad and sprinkle with chooped coriander. Serve hot or cold with a green vegetable.

Cooking Millet ✓

serves 2

GLUTENFREE, DAIRYFREE, EGGFREE, YEASTFREE, FC

I cup (measuring or tea cup) millet
3 cups (as above) water
I tsp cold pressed olive oil

Wash the millet well in a sieve under cold running water. For fluffy millet, boil the water in a pan before adding the millet and simmer gently, covered, for 25–30 minutes. Leave to fluff up, covered, for 10 minutes. Add the oil and stir through the millet. For creamier millet, start the millet in cold water.

Alternatively, cook the millet in a pressure cooker following the instructions for rice, perhaps adding some cauliflower, onion and carrot to cook with the grain for an instant meal.

Cook's note

Millet is the only alkaline grain and therefore recommended for balancing acid/alkaline levels on the diet. Use in any recipe requiring rice or another grain, particularly on Stage 2 of the diet.

Baby Protein Balls ✓

serves 4

GLUTENFREE, DAIRYFREE, EGGFREE, YEASTFREE, FC

---

50 g/2 oz pumpkin, sunflower and linseeds
½ bag sprouted alfalfa
2 celery sticks, finely chopped
I dsp curry powder
4 tsp lemon juice
I dsp yeastfree tamari
2 tbsp chopped parsley
4 tbsp chopped chives

Grind the seeds in a coffee grinder until fine like ground almonds – about 4 pulses.

Add the remaining ingredients except the chives and whizz until smooth.

Roll into small balls and then roll into the chopped chives to coat.

Cook's note
Take these for lunch or as a nutritious snack with some vegetable sticks. Store for a maximum of 3 days in the fridge.

Buckwheat Risotto

serves 4

GLUTENFREE, DAIRYFREE, EGGFREE, YEASTFREE, FC

---

175 g/6 oz buckwheat grains, rinsed
1l/1¾ pts yeastfree vegetable stock
225g/8oz broccoli or calabrese, divided into florets and
with slices of stalk
225 g/8 oz carrots, grated
1 tbsp olive oil
1 tbsp ghee
2 onions, finely chopped
15 g/½ oz dried shitaki mushrooms, soaked according to
instructions on packet
2 tbsp chopped parsley or chervil

Cook the buckwheat in the stock for about 30 minutes. After 20 minutes add the broccoli and carrots and continue cooking. Drain.

Heat the olive oil and ghee and gently fry the onions until translucent. Add the shitaki mushrooms and their soaking liquid, and toss with the onions for 2 minutes. Stir in the buckwheat and vegetables, and chopped herbs. Serve with your favourite green vegetables.

Green Lentils with Spinach, Ginger and Eggs

serves 4

GLUTENFREE, DAIRYFREE, YEASTFREE

200g/7 oz green lentils, soaked overnight
with a strip of kombu
700ml/1 ¼ pts water
3 tbsp olive oil
I tsp grated ginger
bunch of coriander, chopped
450 g/I lb spinach, washed and chopped
6 eggs
salt and pepper
grated rind of I lemon
2tbsp lemon juice

Drain the lentils and kombu and rinse under running water. Combine the lentils, kombu and fresh water in a large pan and bring to the boil. Drain the lentils and kombu again and return to the pan with another 700ml/1¼ pints fresh water. Bring to the boil and simmer gently for about 35 minutes. Drain, reserve the kombu and chop finely.

Heat the wok, add the oil and then the grated ginger. After a few seconds add the coriander and spinach and move around to coat with oil. Stir-fry until the spinach has collapsed and wilted. Add the cooked lentils and chopped kombu, stir well and simmer for 5 minutes.

While this is cooking, hard boil the eggs for 7 minutes, then run cold water on to them until they are cold. Crack the shells, peel and chop finely. Add a pinch of salt and pepper, the lemon rind and juice. Serve the lentil mixture with the chopped eggs and some steamed fish (optional).

Mexican Hummus ✓

serves 4

GLUTENFREE, DAIRYFREE, EGGFREE, YEASTFREE, FC

---

225 g/8 oz chickpeas soaked overnight in 570 ml/I pt water
I medium onion, chopped
3 garlic cloves, chopped
I tbsp cold pressed olive oil
I fresh green chilli (optional)
6 spring onions
Grated rind and juice of I lime
2 ripe tomatoes, skinned and chopped
I tsp cayenne pepper
2 tbsp chopped coriander

Drain the chickpeas of their soaking water and rinse well. Put the chickpeas in a pan, add enough water to cover and bring to the boil. Simmer for 45 minutes, covered, until tender. Drain but reserve some cooking liquid. Transfer the chickpeas to a food processor and purée until creamy and smooth. (You may need to do this in batches depending on size of your processor bowl.) Place three-quarters of the creamed chickpeas in a mixing bowl and leave the rest in the processor. Sauté the onion and garlic in the olive oil until translucent. Process with the remaining chickpea mixture.

Wearing rubber gloves, deseed and chop the chilli. Add to the processor bowl and whizz until tiny green specks of chilli are visible. If the mixture is very dry add a tablespoon or two of the cooking liquid. Stir this mixture into the chickpeas in the mixing bowl.

Trim and finely chop the spring onions and add to the bowl with the grated rind and juice of the lime. Fold in the chopped tomatoes, cayenne pepper and chopped coriander. Season to taste. Leave to stand for an hour or so before serving to allow the flavours to develop.

Cook's note

Alternatively, leave out the tomatoes, chilli and cayenne pepper and flavour with 2–3 tablespoons of light tahini. This will produce a more traditionally flavoured hummus. If you are short of time, tinned chick peas can be used instead of dried.

Spinach, Coriander and Lemon Falafel

serves 4 (makes about 16 small cakes)

GLUTENFREE, DAIRYFREE, EGGFREE, YEASTFREE, FC

---

4 tbsp olive oil
I medium onion, sliced
I garlic clove, chopped
425 g/15 oz organic chickpeas
2 dsp light tahini
I tbsp thawed frozen or leftover spinach
grated rind of I lemon
2 tbsp lemon juice
6 sprigs of coriander

Heat quarter of the oil in a heavy frying pan. Add the onion and garlic and fry until translucent. Do not wash the pan. Drain the chickpeas and place in a food processor with the onion and garlic and all the other ingredients except the rest of the oil, (the spinach must be thawed if using frozen). Process until the mixture forms a smooth, thick green pâté. Turn into a bowl. Take a dessertspoon of the paste and form into small cakes. Heat the remaining oil in a frying pan. Add the cakes and cook in batches, turning once, until they are brown on both sides.

Serve with tahini sauce and lemon or lime wedges and Winter Coleslaw with Sea Vegetables, Mustard and Lemon.

Butterbean, Aubergine and Celeriac Purée   ✓

serves 4

GLUTENFREE, DAIRYFREE, EGGFREE, YEASTFREE, FC

---

225 g/8 oz celeriac, peeled and cubed
1 medium aubergine
1 tbsp olive oil and ghee mixed
1 medium onion, sliced
2 garlic cloves, sliced
1 tsp curry powder
1 tsp ground coriander
1 tsp ground cumin
425 g/15 oz tin butterbeans
1 tsp chopped dill

Heat the grill to its highest setting. While it is heating cover the celeriac with water, add a squeeze of lemon juice and cook for 10–15 minutes, until soft. Drain well and mash. When the grill is hot, roast the aubergine on all sides until brown. Remove and leave to cool.

Heat the oil and ghee in a frying pan. Add the onion and garlic and fry until they just start to turn brown. Add the curry powder, coriander and cumin and sauté the mixture until crusty. Remove from the heat.

Scoop out the aubergine flesh with a metal spoon, dragging down the skin to remove every scrap of pulp. Add to the food processor along with the mashed celeriac, drained butterbeans and the onion, garlic and spice mixture. Run the processor for as long as it takes to make a smooth quite sloppy purée. Turn out into a dish and mix in the dill. Serve as a dipper with pieces of well roasted lamb or grilled chicken, some spring cabbage or greens or on top of Vegetable Pancakes.

Puy Lentils and Courgettes in a Herb Sauce   ✓

serves 4

GLUTENFREE, DAIRYFREE, EGGFREE, YEASTFREE, FC

175g/6oz puy lentils

1.75l/3 pts water

strip of kombu

1 tbsp olive oil

1 large onion, chopped

½ head of celery, chopped

225 g/8 oz courgettes, sliced

110 g/4 oz fresh or frozen peas

275 ml/10 fl oz lentil stock

2 tbsp finely chopped parsley

3 tbsp finely chopped mint

2 tsp chopped oregano

1 bay leaf

2 tsp yeastfree tamari

grated rind of 1 lemon

1 tbsp lemon juice

black pepper

2 tsp finely chopped chives

Wash the lentils and place in a pan. Cover with the water, add the kombu and bring to the boil. Simmer for 35 minutes. Drain, reserve about 275 ml/½ pint of lentil water and remove the kombu. When the kombu is cool, chop into small pieces.

Heat the olive oil in a pan and sauté the onion and celery for 5 minutes until translucent. Add the courgettes, peas and half the cooked lentils. Purée the second half of the lentils in a food processor or blender until smooth and add to the pan. Stir in the lentil stock until you have a thick sauce. Add the parsley, mint, oregano, bay leaf, tamari and lemon rind and juice. Cook for a further 15 minutes. Adjust the seasoning with black pepper, sprinkle with chives and serve. Serve with a green vegetable.

Cook's note
Breaking down half the lentils in the food processor helps digestion of the carbohydrate begun by the enzymes in the kombu.

Black-eyed Bean Stew with Mint

serves 4

GLUTENFREE, DAIRYFREE, EGGFREE, YEASTFREE, FC

**250 g/9 oz black eyed beans and a strip of kombu,
soaked overnight in cold water and drained
I tbsp olive oil
2 medium onions, chopped
3 garlic cloves, sliced
2 carrots, finely chopped
I red pepper
I green chilli, deseeded and finely chopped
I tbsp sesame seeds
I tsp ground cumin
I tsp black mustard seeds
I tsp celery seeds
250 ml/8 fl oz chicken or vegetable stock
5 sprigs of mint, chopped**

Cook the beans and kombu covered, in fresh water for 30 minutes until tender.

Drain the beans and kombu. When the kombu is cool, chop it finely and reserve with the beans.

Heat the olive oil in a heavy pan. Add the onions, garlic and carrots and sauté for 5 minutes until transparent. While this is cooking, char the skin of the red pepper on all sides under a high grill. Set aside to cool.

Add the green chilli, sesame seeds, cumin, mustard and celery seeds, onions and carrots and fry off for 2 mins scraping around the pan as a crust begins to form. Add the chicken or vegetable stock and stir to mix well.

Peel the skin off the red pepper and slice into thin strips. Add to the mixture in the pan along with the black eyed-beans and kombu. This type of bean stew is 'dry'. Of course, if you like it more 'wet' add more stock. Stir in the chopped mint. Serve with green vegetables.

Savoury Nutty Seed Cakes

serves 6

GLUTENFREE, DAIRYFREE, YEASTFREE

110g/4oz walnuts, shelled
110g/4oz almonds, shelled
75g/3oz sunflower seeds
50g/2oz pumpkin seeds
25g/1oz linseeds
1 organic egg, beaten
1 tbsp olive oil
50g/2oz cooked brown rice
2 crushed cardamom seeds (removed from shell)
½ tsp grated ginger
¼ tsp freshly grated nutmeg
3 tbsp chopped parsley
3 tbsp cold pressed olive oil

Process the nuts and seeds through a coffee grinder or blender until finely ground. Place in a bowl and add the remaining ingredients, except the oil. Mix well. Divide into cakes, pressing together with your fingers.

Heat the oil gently in a heavy pan. Add the cakes and fry in batches until brown on both sides. Serve with a green vegetable in the winter or a salad in the summer.

Lentil Burgers ✓

makes 24 small burgers

GLUTENFREE, DAIRYFREE, YEASTFREE, FC

**450 g/1lb brown lentils, soaked overnight
with strip of kombu
2 large onions, finely chopped
2 garlic cloves, crushed
1 large red pepper, chopped small
2 carrots, peeled and chopped small
ghee and olive oil for frying
1 tsp dried thyme
1 tbsp Bragg or yeastfree tamari
1 egg, beaten
1 tbsp chopped parsley
black pepper**

Drain the soaked lentils and kombu, rinse in a sieve and place in a large saucepan with 900 ml/1½ pints of water. Bring them to the boil for 1 minute then drain in a sieve. Cover with 900 ml/ 1½ pints fresh water, bring to the boil and simmer for about 45 minutes. When nearly all the liquid has been absorbed and the lentils squash between finger and thumb, drain the lentils.

While the lentils are cooking, sauté the onions, garlic, red pepper and carrots in the oil and ghee for about 5–7 minutes, until the carrots are done. Add the thyme and tamari and mix well. Transfer to a large bowl. Process half the lentils and kombu until mushy. Add both batches of lentils to the vegetable mixture and stir in the beaten egg and chopped parsley. Now make 24 small burgers by shaping and pressing spoonfuls of the mixture between your hands – don't worry if they look ragged – that's part of their charm. Heat 2 tbs oil and ghee in a large frying pan and fry in batches until golden and crispy on both sides. Serve with a green vegetable.

Fish

Tuna, Broccoli and Celeriac Casserole ✓
serves 2

GLUTENFREE, DAIRYFREE, EGGFREE, YEASTFREE, FC

---

110 g/4 oz broccoli, divided into small florets
200 g/7 oz celeriac or celery, peeled and cubed
1 tbsp Sea Vegetable Seasoning
25 g/1 oz cornflour or arrowroot
1 tbsp oil from tin of tuna, or 1 tbsp olive oil
½ red pepper, chopped
4 spring onions, chopped
1 garlic clove, crushed
200 g/7 oz tin tuna in sunflower or soya oil

Cover the broccoli and celeriac with water and cook for 5 minutes. Drain, but reserve about 275 ml/10 fl oz of the cooking water in a jug. Add the sea vegetable seasoning to the liquid and stir well. Mix a small amount of this stock with the cornflour or arrowroot and blend into a cream in a cup. Return to the jug of stock and stir again.

Heat the oil in a frying pan and fry off the red pepper, spring onions and garlic for 4 minutes. Add the stock and stir constantly until the sauce thickens and comes to the boil. Cook for another minute. Stir in the drained tuna and the reserved broccoli and celeriac. Serve with watercress salad.

Tuna Pâté ✓

serves 4

GLUTENFREE, DAIRYFREE, YEASTFREE, FC

---

200 g/7 oz tin tuna, in oil
4 spring onions, chopped
$\frac{1}{2}$ red pepper, chopped
2 tbsp Mayonnaise (see page 132)
1 tbsp chopped parsley, coriander or dill

Drain the tuna and mash with a fork . Add the chopped spring onions, red pepper, mayonnaise and herbs and mix well. Serve in a lunch box to fill cos lettuce or Chinese leaves, or as a dip with carrot or celery sticks.

Grilled Mackerel with ✓ Coriander and Lime

serves 2

GLUTENFREE, DAIRYFREE, EGGFREE, YEASTFREE, FC

---

2 mackerel, cleaned and gutted
2 limes, 1 quartered, 1 halved
4 sprigs of coriander
sea salt and black pepper

Preheat the grill to its highest setting and oil the grid.

Wipe the mackerel with kitchen paper and place a couple of lime quarters and 2 sprigs of coriander inside each one. Grind a little sea salt, mix with black pepper and add to the cavity. Make four diagonal slashes on each side of each mackerel with a very sharp knife.

Arrange the fish on the grid, reduce the grill to medium for about and cook 6 minutes on each side. Serve with the lime halves, and some puréed spinach or other strong flavoured green vegetable such as Swiss chard.

Fillet of Trout on a Bed of Leeks, Courgettes and Watercress

serves 4

GLUTENFREE, DAIRYFREE, EGGFREE, YEASTFREE

---

4 trout fillets, skinned

3 tbsp bottled water

3 tbsp raw, unfilled cider vinegar

40 g/1 ½ oz butter or mixed ghee and olive oil

½ tsp dried tarragon

4 leeks

4 courgettes

2 tsp cornflour

½ bunch of watercress, chopped

grated rind of 1 lemon

125 g/4 ½ oz live plain yoghurt

black pepper

Preheat the oven to 180°C/350°F/Gas Mark 4.

Roll up the trout fillets and place them in an overproof dish. Pour over the bottled water and cider vinegar. Dot with half the butter or ghee and olive oil and the dried tarragon. Cover with foil cook on high for 20 minutes. Set aside to cool. Trim the leeks, then cut across each one to make three or four sections. Slice very finely down the length of each section and rinse well. Grate the courgettes.

Melt the remaining butter in a pan and sauté the leeks and courgettes for 2–3 minutes until soft, stirring constantly. Add the cornflour and cook for 1 minute, stirring constantly. Add the chopped watercress and lemon rind and mix through the vegetables. Reduce the heat and beat in the yoghurt and any stock from the dish the fish was cooked in. Cook for a few minutes until the mixture begins to thicken, then continue to cook for a further 1 minute.

Spoon into serving dish and place the rolled fish fillets on top. Reheat in the oven for 20 minutes.

Marinated Rainbow Trout Salad   ✓

serves 1–2

GLUTENFREE, DAIRYFREE, EGGFREE, YEASTFREE, FC

I rainbow trout, filleted or 2 trout fillets
juice of I lemon
2 tbsp olive oil
2 sprigs of dill or I tsp dried dill
strips of lemon rind
I tbsp chopped chives
black pepper

Place the fish in a shallow dish and pour over the lemon juice and olive oil. Break up the sprigs of dill and tuck under the fish with the lemon rind, or scatter over the dried dill. Cover and put in the fridge for 8 hours or overnight, turning two or three times.

Preheat the grill to its highest setting.

Brush the grid with oil and arrange the trout evenly, discarding the dill and lemon strips. Reduce the heat to medium and grill for 4 minutes on each side, or until the flesh of the trout is opaque and cooked. Serve hot, immediately garnished with chopped chives and black pepper or cold, broken into flakes with a salad of mixed leaves or celeriac rosti.

Oat and Lemon Crusted Fish

serves 1

DAIRYFREE, EGGFREE, YEASTFREE

I tbsp organic oats
grated rind of I lemon
I tbsp Sea Vegetable Seasoning
about I 10 g/4 oz oily fish fillets, such as herring or mackerel

---

Mix all the ingredients except the fish together and put on to a plate. Press the fish into the mixture so that the fillet surface is covered.

Heat the grill to its highest setting.

Oil the grill grid and arrange the fillets on the grid. Grill for 4 minutes on high, then reduce to medium. Turn the fish and continue cooking for another 5–6 minutes. Turn off the grill and leave the fish to rest for 2 minutes before serving.

Sardine Crackers   ✓

serves 4

GLUTENFREE, DAIRYFREE, EGGFREE, YEASTFREE, FC

---

8 fresh sardines, gutted
8 lemon slices, halved
8 sprigs of dill
I lemon, quartered

Preheat the oven to 190°C/375°F/Gas mark 5.

Wash the sardines and pat dry. For each sardine prepare a sheet of baking parchment or greaseproof paper about three times its own size. Place a sardine parallel with the long side, about 2 inches from the end. Tuck half lemon slices inside each sardine with a sprig of dill. Roll up the sardine very loosely and twist the paper ends like a cracker. Place on a baking tray and bake in the oven for 35 minutes.

Remove from the oven and carefully (the cracker will be hot) untwist the paper to open the sardine. Lift on to individual plates and slide out the sardines and juice on to the plates.

Serve with a watercress garnish and a green vegetable.

Cook's note
Sardines are excellent fish for the *Beat Candida Diet* being high in omega 3 fatty acids. This cooking method keeps the smell of cooking fish to a minimum and retains all the nutritional fish juices.

Haddock, Coconut, Lemon and Parsley Kedgeree

serves 4

GLUTENFREE, DAIRYFREE, EGGFREE, YEASTFREE

---

550 g/1¼ lb fresh haddock, cod or other
thick fleshed white fish
grated rind and juice of 1 lemon
2 fl oz/50 ml bottled water
40 g/1½ oz butter, ghee or olive oil
black pepper
1 medium onion, finely chopped
3 garlic cloves, sliced
1 tsp ground cumin
1 dsp ground coriander
1 dsp turmeric
1 tbsp curry powder
2 tbsp cornflour
275 ml/10 fl oz coconut milk
50g/2oz coarsely chopped whole almonds
3 tbsp chopped parsley
sea salt and black pepper

Pre-heat the oven to 180°C/350°F/Gas Mark 4.

Place the fish in a microwave dish. Add the lemon juice and water, dot with the butter and add a couple of turns of black pepper. Cover and bake for 20 minutes. Drain the cooking liquid from the fish and place in a heavy pan; flake the fish and reserve.

Sauté the onion and garlic in the fish liquid until soft. Add the cumin, coriander, turmeric and curry powder and fry for 3 minutes to blend the flavours. Stir in the cornflour and scrape around the pan to mix and cook until the sauce thickens. Reduce the heat to a simmer and add the flaked fish and chopped parsley. Lightly season with sea salt and black pepper. Serve with a broccoli and spinach salad or brown rice.

Fish in a Parcel with Nutty Vegetable Shreds

serves 1

GLUTENFREE, DAIRYFREE, EGGFREE, YEASTFREE, FC

This recipe is exciting enough for all your friends to enjoy when they come to dinner. For each person you need:

---

2 tsp sesame seeds
I dsp sesame oil
I dsp yeastfree tamari
15 ml/I tbsp flaked almonds
I small garlic clove
I fillet of bream, salmon, trout or other firm fish
1/4 leek, finely shredded
I carrot, peeled and finely shredded
some fine shreds of root ginger and lemon grass
sesame oil, for brushing

Preheat the oven to 190°C/375°F/Gas Mark 5.

If you have a coffee grinder, grind half the sesame seeds up first in this - about 6 pulses. Then, place the sesame oil, tamari, ground or whole sesame seeds, almonds and garlic in a food processor and whizz until well blended. Scrape on to a plate and lay the fish, skin up, on top of this marinade. Leave aside. Cut out squares of baking parchment the width of the roll for each portion – minimum size 30.5 cm/12 in square. If you don't have paper large enough cut the right sized square out of foil and line with baking parchment. Brush the paper with sesame oil.

Take the fish fillet from the marinade and place, right side up, in the centre of the paper. Top with the vegetable shreds and the remaining sesame seeds. Drizzle some of the marinade over. Pull up the long sides of the paper and staple together, then pull up each end and staple to the first join to make a sealed parcel. Lift on to a baking tray lined with foil to catch any escaping juices from the parcel, put into the oven and cook for 25 minutes. Remove from the oven.

Cut open the parcel and slide the contents on to a warm serving plate, tipping the juices over the fish, plus any that have leaked on to the foil. Serve with a fragrant pilau rice with mange-touts, grated lime and ginger, or a celeriac rosti, if you are food combining.

Thai Fishcakes with Coriander ✓

serves 4 (makes 12 cakes)

GLUTENFREE, DAIRYFREE, EGGFREE, YEASTFREE, FC

450g/1lb firm fish, such as cod, haddock, salmon or trout
4 spring onions, chopped
4 celery sticks, chopped
6 sprigs of coriander, roughly chopped
2 tbsp Thai Green Curry Paste
rind and juice of 1 lime
2 tbsp olive oil

Skin the fish and search for any bones and remove. Place all the ingredients except the olive oil in a blender or food processor and blend until just smooth. Scrape out into a mixing bowl. Take tablespoonfuls of the mixture and form them into balls, loosely rolling them between your hands. Place in the centre of a plate and press down to form cakes. As you make up the 12 cakes store them, covered, in the fridge for an hour, or place them in the freezer for 30 minutes.

Heat the oil gently in a heavy frying pan and fry the cakes in batches, about four at a time, turning once, until they are golden brown.

Serve with Celery, Cucumber and Red Onion Salsa and a green vegetable or salad.

Poached Salmon with Herbs ✓

serves 4

GLUTENFREE, DAIRYFREE, EGGFREE, YEASTFREE, FC

½ leek, chopped into thin strips
½ lemon, cut into 4 slices
½ tsp dried tarragon or dried dill
4 salmon steaks or fillets (skinned), about 4 oz each
I tbsp lemon juice
125 ml/4 fl oz vegetable stock or homemade fish stock
I lemon, cut into 4 slices, to garnish
watercress sprigs, to garnish

Arrange the leek strips, the half lemon slices and half the dried herbs in a large frying pan and top with the salmon. Mix the lemon juice and stock together and pour over the fish. Sprinkle with the remaining herbs. Bring the liquid to the boil then simmer very gently, without covering, for 6 minutes, or until the fish is cooked through.

Lift the fish out with a fish slice and let it drain for a few seconds before arranging on individual plates. Garnish with the slices of lemon and watercress sprigs and serve with another green vegetable.

Chicken, lamb and game

Marinated Roast Chicken with Garlic and Mustard Seeds ✓

serves 4

GLUTENFREE, DAIRYFREE, EGGFREE, YEASTFREE, FC

---

2 tbsp olive oil
6 garlic cloves, crushed
I dsp mustard seeds
3 tbsp chicken or vegetable stock
I dsp cider vinegar
4 sprigs of rosemary or I dsp dried rosemary
I medium organic chicken

Preheat the oven to 220°C, 425°F, Gas mark 7

Process the oil, garlic, mustard seeds, stock and cider vinegar in a blender or food processor until the garlic is broken down. Rub this marinade all over the chicken. Tuck the rosemary inside the chicken or pat over the dried rosemary. Leave in the fridge for 8 hours or overnight, turning the chicken at least once.

Remove the chicken from the marinade, reserving any liquid for basting.

Turn the chicken breast side down and place in a baking tin. Roast for 20 minutes. Turn breast side up, baste with the remaining marinade and cook for a further 20 minutes. reduce the heat to 190°C/375°F/Gas mark 5 and roast for a further 30 minutes. To check the chicken is done, stick a sharp knife into the thickest part of the thigh – the juice must run clear. If the juice runs pink or red, continue cooking until it runs clear.

Serve with your favourite vegetables, taking a high ratio of vegetables to chicken.

Cook's note

This method of cooking the bird upside down to begin with is excellent for all poultry and game ensuring the cooking juices run down into the breast meat to prevent drying out.

Unsuitable at stage 2 if you add potatoes or a grain to this meal.

Chinese Chicken Salad   ✓

serves 4

GLUTENFREE, DAIRYFREE, EGGFREE, YEASTFREE, FC

2–3 chicken breasts
2 garlic cloves, halved
35 oz/12 oz bag of young spinach
2 tbsp olive oil
1 tsp sesame oil
juice of 1 lemon
1 tbsp yeastfree tamari
knob of root ginger, peeled and chopped
25g/1oz pumpkin seeds

Preheat the oven to 200°C/400°F/Gas Mark.

Arrange the chicken breasts in the middle of a large sheet of baking parchment or greaseproof paper and scatter over the garlic. Bring the long sides together, fold over once and staple to seal, leaving room around the chicken. Bake for 40 minutes in the oven. Remove the stalks from the spinach and wash well. Shake off the excess water.

While the chicken is cooking heat the wok. Add half the olive oil then the spinach, pushing down with a wooden spoon. Toss the spinach around until it has wilted.

Remove the chicken from the oven and carefully undo the parcel without losing the juices. Tear or slice the chicken into thin strips, mix with the wilted spinach and cooking juices and pile on a serving dish.

Make a dressing from the remaining ingredients, including the remaining olive oil, and pour over the chicken and spinach, tossing through the salad to coat. Serve with Grated Carrot and Sesame Seed Salad.

Grilled Chicken Pieces ✓

serves 2

GLUTENFREE, DAIRYFREE, EGGFREE, YEASTFREE, FC

**3 garlic cloves, chopped
1 tsp dried tarragon or other herb
rind and juice of 1 lemon
1 tbsp olive oil
125 ml/4 fl oz chicken stock
2 chicken pieces**

Process the first five ingredients until well blended. Pour over the chicken, turning through the marinade, and place, covered, in the fridge for a minimum of 15 minutes or a maximum of 8 hours, turning the chicken once or twice.

Preheat the grill to its highest setting.

Oil the grill grid and arrange the chicken pieces on the grill. Drizzle over a little of the marinating mixture. Cook for 10 minutes on each side, or until the chicken is cooked through.

Serve with green vegetables, baked onions or Celery, Cucumber and Red Onion Salsa or Mediterranean Onion Salad.

Cook's note

A marinade for meat or fish containing lemon juice starts the digestion process for you as the acid juice tenderises the surface protein. However, too long a marinade will spoil the texture of the meat so a maximum of 8 hours is recommended.

Creamy Coconut Chicken with ✓ Almonds and Coriander

serves 4–6

GLUTENFREE, DAIRYFREE, EGGFREE, YEASTFREE, FC

I tsp cumin seeds
I tsp coriander seeds
I tsp mustard seeds
I tsp turmeric
knob of root ginger, peeled and grated
4 garlic cloves, crushed
75 ml/3 fl oz live plain yoghurt
I chicken, jointed into 6 pieces, or 6–8 chicken pieces
2 tbsp olive oil and ghee
I medium onion, peeled and sliced
225 ml/8 fl oz coconut milk
25 g/I oz ground almonds
handful of chopped coriander
slices of lime

Dry roast the three seeds in a frying pan over low heat for 2 minutes, until the mustard seeds pop. Add the turmeric. Cool down then grind in a pestle and mortar or coffee grinder until fine and powdery. Mix with the ginger, garlic and yoghurt, and rub over the chicken pieces.

Heat the oil and ghee in a heavy frying pan and cook the onion until translucent. Add the chicken pieces and the rest of the marinade and cook until the chicken browns. Stir in the coconut milk and ground almonds and continue cooking for another 25 minutes. Stir in the chopped coriander just before serving. Serve with slices of lime and lots of green vegetables, and with some rice for guests who may not be food combining.

Indian Chicken Stir-fry

serves 4

GLUTENFREE, DAIRYFREE, YEASTFREE, FC

225g/8oz boneless chicken breast, skinned
1 egg white
1 tsp cornflour
2 tbs olive oil and ghee mixed
175g/6oz red peppers, deseeded & cubed
70ml/2½ fl oz chicken stock
2 tsp curry powder
1 tsp cider vinegar
1 tbsp yeastfree tamari
1 tsp cornflour blended with 1 tsp water

Cut the chicken breast into thin strips, slicing with the grain. Mix the egg white and cornflour in a bowl, add the chicken strips and toss them until well coated. Cover and place in the fridge for 10 mins.

Heat the wok. Add half the oil and ghee mix, then the chicken mixture and stir fry very quickly to prevent it sticking until white, about 4 minutes. Remove the chicken and set aside on kitchen paper. Drain off any remaining oil and ghee and discard and wipe out the wok.

Heat the remaining oil and ghee in the wok and add the peppers, stir frying for about 2 minutes. Stir in the remaining ingredients, except the chicken, and cook for a further 2 minutes. Add the chicken strips and coat with the sauce. Serve immediately with a green vegetable.

Pheasant Casserole with Celery ✓
and Baby Onions

serves 4

GLUTENFREE, DAIRYFREE, EGGFREE, YEASTFREE

---

1 onion
1 small sharp cooking apple stuck with 4 cloves
2 sprigs of sage
1 pheasant
4 tbsp olive oil
1 head of celery
12 pickling onions
1 tbsp cider vinegar
275ml/10 fl oz chicken or yeastfree vegetable stock
1–2 tbsp cornflour
bunch of watercress

Preheat the oven to 200°C/400°F/Gas Mark 6.

The onion, cooking apple stuck with cloves and sage sprigs go inside the cavity of the bird, so depending on the size of the pheasant you may need to halve or quarter the onion and apple to fit the cavity. When the bird is stuffed, brush it with 3 table-spoons of oil and place it, breast down, in a baking tin. It does not matter if it falls to one side. Roast in the oven for 20 minutes.

While it is cooking, chop the head of celery into chunks and rinse off any dirt. Peel the pickling onions by blanching in boiling water for 3 minutes which makes the skins slip off more easily.

Take the pheasant out of the oven and distribute the onions and celery around the bird, drizzling over the remaining oil. Continue cooking for the rest of the first 20 minute period. When this time is up, remove the tin from the oven, turn the pheasant breast side up and turn the vegetables over in the cooking juices. Add the cider vinegar to the stock and pour around the pheasant. Cook for a further 50 minutes, basting the pheasant occasionally with the stock.

Turn off the heat, but leave the pheasant in the oven. Mix the cornflour with 1-2 tbsp water to a cream. Take the pheasant out of the oven and remove the onion and apple which will by now be very soft. Discard the apple and sage sprigs, and place the onion in the food processor or blender. Lift out the vegetables from the baking tin, arrange around the pheasant and return to the oven to keep warm.

Add some stock from the vegetables to the processor and whizz until smooth. Pour into a small pan with the remaining stock and the slaked cornflour. Stir well to mix, then heat very gently, stirring constantly, until the gravy thickens and looks glossy. Bring the pheasant out of the oven and carve. Serve with the celery and onion in gravy, garnished with watercress.

Cook's note
Stuffing the cavity of poultry and game and cooking the bird breast down for the whole or part of the cooking time helps to flavour and moisten the meat.

Lamb Chops with Avocado Salsa   ✓

serves 4

GLUTENFREE, DAIRYFREE, EGGFREE, YEASTFREE, FC

I lime
I lamb chop per person, or use a chicken piece,
salmon or trout fillet

Avocado salsa:
grated rind of I lime
1/4 cucumber, peeled and diced
4 spring onions, finely chopped
I garlic clove, crushed
I avocado, peeled and finely diced
handful of fresh coriander, chopped
I dsp yeastfree tamari

Grate the lime and set aside. Squeeze out the lime juice and pour over the lamb, chicken or fish. Set aside for 15 mins while you make the salsa.

To make the salsa, mix all the ingredients together and add the grated lime rind. Cover and store in the fridge.

Heat the grill to its highest setting.

Oil the grid and set the chops on the grill pan. Sear for 2 minutes. Reduce the heat to moderate and continue cooking, turning once, until well done, about 6–8 minutes each side depending upon the thickness of the meat. Chicken breasts or pieces will need 10–12 minutes each side; fish will need 5–6 minutes each side.

Serve with dollops of avocado salsa and a green vegetable.

Marinated Lamb Kebabs   ✓

serves 4

GLUTENFREE, DAIRY FREE, EGGFREE, YEASTFREE, FC

½ portion of Lemon and Garlic Sauce leaving out the dill
sprigs of rosemary
275g/10oz fillet of lamb or leg of lamb
16 pickling onions
1 red pepper
1 medium aubergine
12 cherry tomatoes
16 fat garlic cloves, unpeeled (optional)

The night before, or at least 4–8 hours before cooking, prepare the Lemon and Garlic Sauce leaving out the chopped dill and adding sprigs of rosemary or 2 tbsp dried rosemary instead to the marinade. Cut the lamb fillet into small even-sized chunks about 3.5cm/1½ in square. If you use leg of lamb do the same but try to cut around the silvery sinew or keep it to the inside of the chunks, and trim of any large pieces of fat – a little fat will be useful to keep the meat moist and well flavoured so don't go overboard about removing every vestige of it.

Skin the onions by blanching them in boiling water for 3 minutes and then draining – the skins should slip off more easily this way. Cut the red pepper into chunks larger than the meat and take out the seeds. Cut the aubergine into similar sized chunks as the meat and separate the fat garlic cloves but do not peel, if using.

Place all the ingredients in a bowl, pour on the marinade and turn everything over several times to coat with the marinade. Cover and set aside in the fridge for at least 4 hours. If possible, turn the ingredients over several times before cooking.

Just before cooking, preheat the grill to its highest setting and thread the ingredients on to 4 large or 8 small metal or bamboo skewers, alternating the meat, onions, pepper, aubergine and garlic cloves, allowing a little space between each item. Brush with the remaining marinade and reserve the rest.

Reduce the grill to medium. Cook, turning the skewers every few minutes using an oven glove as they may be very hot, and basting with the remaining marinade to allow the kebabs to brown gently till the meat is tender - about 15–20 minutes in all.

Serve with Mediterranean Onion Salad and mixed salad leaves, or with any green vegetable or stir-fried vegetables such as Mange-tout, Asparagus and Spring Onion Stir-fry.

Alternatively, the kebabs may be cooked on a barbecue but if you do so make sure you can control the heat and flames – burnt meat and vegetables are difficult to digest apart from being unpleasant to eat.

Pancakes

Indian Dhal Pancakes ✓

makes about 10 pancakes

GLUTENFREE, DAIRYFREE, EGGFREE, YEASTFREE, FC

---

200 g/7 oz red lentils
50 g/2 oz frozen peas, thawed
small cube of ginger, peeled and grated
2 garlic cloves, peeled
¼ tsp turmeric
½ tsp ground cumin
½ tsp ground coriander
75 ml/3 fl oz water
I small onion, grated
2 tbsp chopped coriander
¼ tsp baking powder
ghee for frying.

Soak the red lentils in 1 litre/1¾ pts) water overnight or for 4 hours, and drain. Drop the peas into boiling water for 3–4 minutes and drain. Combine the peas, ginger, garlic, turmeric, cumin, coriander, lentils and water in a processor and whizz until the mixture makes a smooth batter. Combine the batter with the onion and chopped coriander. Leave covered in the fridge for anything up to 36 hours. Add the baking powder and stir well.

Brush a non-stick frying pan with melted ghee and heat over medium heat. Pour a blob of batter into the centre of the pan, tipping the pan to run the batter out into a thin pancake. Cover and cook for 2 minutes, then turn over until the underside has red spots.

Cook's notes

This is best eaten fresh with scrambled eggs (stages 1 and 3 only) at breakfast, or with vegetable curries.

Savoury Vegetable Pancakes

makes 8–10

GLUTENFREE, DAIRYFREE, YEASTFREE

25g/1oz millet flakes
25g/1oz rice flakes
50g/2oz gram (chickpea) flour
1 organic or free range egg
400 ml/¾ pt goat, rice or oat milk
50g/2oz grated carrot
2 spring onions, finely chopped
1 tbsp curry powder (optional)
olive oil for frying

Mix the flakes and flour together in a large jug. Beat the egg with the chosen milk and add to the dry ingredients, beating together to make a thick batter. Add the carrot, spring onions and curry powder and stir through the batter.

Preheat the oven to its lowest setting.

Pour some olive oil into a cup and brush a thick frying pan with a little of it. Heat the pan and pour about a tablespoonful of batter into the pan. Cook for about 3 minutes then flip over with a fish slice. Depending on the size of the pan and the pancake, you may be able to fry two or three at once. Cook for a further 2 minutes until browned evenly on both sides. Slide on to a plate and stack them up. Keep warm in the oven.

Serve topped with Butterbean, Aubergine and Celeriac Purée and with a salad of lettuce, watercress, carrot and cucumber dressed with Garlic and Cardamom Dressing.

Pudlas (Gujarati Pancakes)   ✓

makes 8

GLUTENFREE, DAIRYFREE, EGGFREE, YEASTFREE, FC

---

225 g/8 oz gram (chickpea) flour
1/2 tsp cayenne pepper
1 tsp cumin seeds, roasted
1/2 tsp sea salt
1/4 tsp turmeric
4 spring onions
110g/4oz frozen peas, thawed
2 tbsp chopped coriander
ghee for frying

Sift the flour into a large bowl, add the remaining ingredients then beat in 300ml/12 fl oz cold water to make a thick batter. Set aside for 15 minutes.

Brush a non-stick frying pan (about 18cm/7 in) with melted ghee. Heat until very hot then pour in a spoonful of batter, tipping the pan to coat evenly. Cook for about 1½ minutes, turn over and cook for a further minute.

Occasional treats

Cheesy Muffins

makes 8–10

GLUTENFREE, DAIRYFREE, YEASTFREE, NO ADDED SUGAR

50 g/2 oz rice flakes
70 g/2½ oz cornmeal
70 g/2½ oz potato flour
2 tbsp sesame seeds
1 dsp baking powder
50 g/2 oz dairyfree margarine (non-hydrogenated)
1 organic or free range egg
300 ml/12 fl oz milk, goat, rice, soya or oat
110 g/4 oz soft goat's cheese
2 spring onions, chopped

Preheat the oven to 200°C/400°F/Gas Mark 6.

Mix all the dry ingredients together. Rub in the margarine. Beat the egg into the chosen milk. Add the cheese and spring onions to the dry mixture, pour on the egg and milk and mix well. Spoon into paper muffin cases and bake for 20–25 minutes until brown and crusty. Serve warm.

Delicious for Sunday brunch with soup, or for a packed lunch with salad or oven roasted vegetables.

Banana Bread

makes 450g / 1lb loaf

GLUTENFREE, YEASTFREE

---

75 g/3 oz creamed coconut from a block
I large banana, sliced
50g/2oz ground almonds
I organic egg
150ml/5fl oz live plain yoghurt
110g/4oz brown rice flour
25g/1oz cornflour
I tsp glutenfree baking powder
I tsp pure vanilla essence

Preheat the oven to 180°C/350°F/Gas Mark 4. Line a 450 g/ 1 lb loaf tin with baking parchment.

If the creamed coconut block is very hard, soften by running hot water over it, or immerse the block in a jug of very hot water for 1 minute. Add the sliced banana, creamed coconut, ground almonds, egg and yoghurt to the bowl of a food processor and whizz to mix all the ingredients together to a smooth cream.

Mix the flours and baking powder in a mixing bowl and stir in the cream from the food processor. Add the vanilla essence and beat until smooth.

Spoon into the lined loaf tin and bake for 30–45 minutes. Test for doneness by inserting a sharp knife into the centre of the loaf – it should be sticky but not wet. Leave the loaf to cool before slicing.

Cook's note
Glutenfree breads and cakes do not keep well so store the banana loaf in the fridge or freeze slices to bring out when you need them.

Orchard Nectar

serves 4

GLUTENFREE, DAIRYFREE, EGGFREE, YEASTFREE

---

900 g/2 lb cooking apples, peeled, cored and thinly sliced
150–250 ml/5–8 fl oz water
8 cloves
I tbsp apple concentrate, apple juice or honey (optional)
grated rind of I unwaxed or organic lemon

Cook the sliced apples in the water with the cloves over high heat until they begin to break down. Reduce the heat and simmer until the apples are soft and fluffy. If using the apple concentrate or honey, add to the apples and stir well. Stir in the grated lemon rind.

You can remove the cloves at this point – best done with a pair of tongs as the apple will be hot. Cool and store in the fridge. Serve with live yoghurt or on its own.

Glutenfree Pastry

GLUTENFREE, DAIRYFREE, YEASTFREE

---

100 g/3½ oz ground almonds
100 g/3½ oz brown rice flour
50 g/2 oz cornflour
100 g/3½ oz non-hydrogenated dairyfree margarine
I organic or free range egg

Preheat the oven to 190°C/375°F/Gas Mark 5.

Place all the ingredients in the food processor and whizz until a ball of dough forms. Chill in the fridge or freeze until required.

Cook's note
Glutenfree pastry is brittle and difficult to handle. To use, chill the pastry. Roll out between sheets of baking parchment or greaseproof paper, cut out and lift, with a fish slice or spatula, into patty tins. It is not suitable for large pastry lids as it is too fragile, but can be pressed into a flan tin for the base of a tart or flan.

Almond, Garlic and Parsley Crumble Topping

serves 4

GLUTENFREE, DAIRYFREE, EGGFREE, YEASTFREE

---

2 tbsp chopped parsley
1 large garlic clove, grated
100 g/3½ oz ground almonds
150 g/5 oz brown rice flour
100 g/3½ oz non-hydrogenated dairyfree margarine

Preheat the oven to 350°F/180°C/Gas Mark 6.

Whizz the parsley in the food processor until roughly chopped. Add the grated garlic and all the other ingredients to the parsley and blend until crumbs form. Alternatively, mix by hand rubbing the margarine into the dry ingredients until crumbs form.

Scatter over Italian Vegetable Salad, and cook for 25–30 minutes. Serve with a green salad dressed Lemon and Garlic Sauce.

Bibliography

'A Clinical Ecology Programme for Assessment and Treatment of Suspected Amalgam Compromised Patients', Dr Alan Hibberd, BioMED Newsletter, No 12

A Matter of Life: The Springhill Centre's holistic approach to caring and healing, Dr Nadia Coates and Norman Jollyman, Optima, 1990 (out of print).

A World Without AIDS, Leon Chaitow and Simon Martin, Thorsons, 1989.

All Day Energy, Kathryn Marsden, Bantam, 1995.

Beat Candida, Gill Jacobs, Vermilion, 1996.

The Bitter Pill, Dr Ellen Grant, Corgi, 1985.

The Body Ecology Diet, Donna Gates and Linda Schatz, BED Publications, 1995.

Breaking the Vicious Cycle: Intestinal Health Through Diet, Elaine Gottschall, The Kirkton Press, 1996.

The Canary and Chronic Fatigue, Dr Majid Ali, Lifespan Press, 1994.

Candida Albicans, Could Yeast Be Your Problem?, Leon Chaitow, Thorsons.

The Complete Candida Yeast Guidebook, Jeanne Marie Martin, with Zolta Rona, Prima Publishing, 1996.

Fats, Nutrition and Health, Robert Erdmann and Meirion Jones, Thorsons, 1990 (out of print).

Fit for Life, Harvey and Marilyn Diamond, Bantam, 1995.

The Food Combining Diet, Kathryn Marsden, Thorsons, 1993.

Food Combining For Health, Doris Grant and Jean Joice, Thorsons, 1993.

Food Combiners' Meal Planner, Kathryn Marsden, Thorsons.

The Food Factor, Barbara Griggs, Penguin, 1988.

Foods that Harm, Foods that Heal, Readers Digest, 1996.

The Foods We Eat, Joanna Blythman, Michael Joseph, 1996.

The HEA Guide to Complementary Medicine and Therapies, Anne Woodham, Health Education Authority, 1994.

The Lactic Acid Bacteria and their Role in Human Health, Dr Nigel Plummer, 1995, BioMED Books.

Macrobiotic Cooking, Aveline Kushi, Warner Books, 1985.

The Missing Diagnosis, Dr Orian Truss, 1985.

On Food and Cooking – The Science and Lore of the Kitchen, Harold McGee, Harper Collins, 1991.

The Practical Guide to Candida (including the UK Directory of Complementary Practitioners who treat Candida albicans holistically) Jane McWhirter, All Hallows House Foundation, £7.50 + £1.50 p&p from Green Library, 6, Rickett Street, London SW6 1RU (Cheques payable to AHHF Candida book).

Principles of Kinesiology, Maggie La Tourelle and Anthea Courtenay, Thorsons, 1997.

Practically Macrobiotic, Keith Michell, Thorsons 1987.

Raw Energy, Leslie Kenton and Susannah Kenton, Vermilion, 1996.

Superbug – Nature's Revenge: Why antibiotics can breed disease, Geoffrey Cannon, Virgin, 1995.

Vegetable Cook Book, Colin Spencer, Conran Octopus, 1995.

The Yeast Connection, Dr William Crook.

Information, support and advice

Action for ME and Chronic Fatigue
PO Box 1302
Wells
Somerset BA5 2WE
Tel: 01749 670799

Membership organisation and charity, £15 a year, for those with ME and candida related problems, and includes access to their Therapy and Information Helpline and a Counselling Helpline. Therapy factsheets are also available on request. Mail order supplements for candida, some at reduced prices for members. Limited number of organic vegetable box schemes available. Publishers of the journal *InterAction*.

The Candida Support Network
All Hallows House Foundation
All Hallows Centre for Natural Health and Healing
Idol Lane
London EC3 5DD

Send a large SAE with a cheque for £5. In return the names and telephone numbers of other network members in your area will be sent to you. Advice on how to set up a support group is also sent.

Candida Workshops UK
10 Burghley Road
London NW5 1UE
0207 428 9577
www.candidaworkshops.co.uk

Gill Jacobs and Jane McWhirter have made a three hour video, *Clear from Candida*. Nutritionist and lecturer, Gillian Hamer, talks about what candida is and what to do about it, Jane McWhirter does an hour's cookery demonstration, and Gill Jacobs talks about stress and the emotions, with contributions from workshop participants. The video comes with a free recipe booklet and costs £19.99 plus £1.50 p&p from Safe Remedies, see below. Candida Workshops also sells mail order books on candida and gut dysbiosis, and runs conferences for health practitioners. Cassettes of the conference lectures are £7.00 each (includes Live Blood Analysis, Dr Sherry Rogers). Visit the web site for listings, up-to-date information and fact-sheets.

Hyperactive Children's Support Group
71 Whyke Lane
Chichester
West Sussex PO21 2DE

Wide experience of treating and helping children with candidiasis. Send an SAE for information.

Candida and Dysbiosis Information Foundation
PO Drawer JF
College Station
TX 774841–5146
USA
Tel: 409 694–8687

The National Candida Society
PO Box 151
Orpington
Kent BR5 1UJ
www.candida-society.org.uk

Run by Dr Christine Tomlinson, an ex sufferer. For £15 a year this group provides a free telephone helpline, and a quarterly newsletter. Local groups are encouraged and supported. £25 vouchers off supplements on joining. Send a large SAE with cheque.

Safe Remedies
144 High Street
Dunbar
East Lothian
Scotland EH42 1JJ
Tel: 01368 864 834
www.saferemedies.co.uk

This company imports excellent products from Australia, especially their Organic Green Barley powder to oxygenate the blood, Olive Leaf Extract, a natural antibiotic and antifungal. Don Chisolm who started this company also imports Live Blood Microscopy equipment, and runs training courses for practitioners.

Finding a practitioner

For a UK Directory of Complementary Practitioners who treat candida albicans holistically, see *The Practical Guide to Candida*, Jane McWhirter, All Hallows House Foundation (see Bibliography).

Bioenergy Healer
Trond Bjornstad
c/o Gill Jacobs
10 Burghley Road
London NW5 1UE
Tel: 0207 428 9577
www.moxifoundation.org

British Homoeopathic Association
27 Devonshire Street
London W1N 1RJ
Tel 0171 935 2163

Members are medically trained practitioners. Send SAE for information and list of members.

Council for Complementary and Alternative Medicine (CCAM)
Park House, Suite D
206–208 Latimer Road
London W10 6RE
Tel 0181 968 3862
Fax 0181 968 3469

Colonics International Association
16 New England Lane
London NW3 4TG
Tel: 0171 483 1595

Institute for Complementary Medicine
PO Box 194

London SE16 1QZ
Tel 0171 237 5165
Fax 0171 237 5175

The Institute holds a general register of practitioners. Send an SAE for a copy.

International Academy of Oral Medicine and Toxicology
72 Harley Street
London W1N 1AE
Tel: 0171 580 3168

National Institute of Medical Herbalists
9 Palace Gate
Exeter
Devon EX1 1JA

Society for the Promotion of Nutritional Therapy
PO Box 47
Heathfield
East Sussex TN21 8ZX
Tel: 01435 867 007
Fax: 01435 868 033

Send SAE for an approved list of practitioners.

Society of Homoeopaths
2 Artizan Road
Northampton
Northamptonshire NN1 4HU
Tel: 01604 21400

Registers non-medically qualified homoeopaths who completed a four year training course followed by one year clinical supervision. Send SAE for list of members.

Tests

Biolab Medical Unit
9 Weymouth Street

London W1N 3FF
Tel: 0171 636 5959

Gut fermentation test, Intestinal permeability (leaky gut) test, Low blood sugar test. Only through a doctor's referral.

E.P. UK
25 New Road
Spalding
Lincs PE11 1DQ

Litmus paper for home testing of acid/alkaline balance (pH levels).

Parascope
Department of Microbiology
Chapel Allerton Hospital
Chapeltown Road
Leeds LS7 4SA
Tel: 0113 2924657

Testing for chronic gut parasites using stool specimens. Doctor's referral needed.

Courses and tapes

Clinically Standardized Meditation (Tapes and Manuals)
PO Box 2280
Bournmouth
Dorset BH9 2ZE
Tel: 01202 518968
Fax: 01202 547444

Learning for Life Ltd
(Clinically Standardised Meditation Tapes)
The Coach House
Chinewood Manor
32 Manor Road
Bournemouth BH1 3EZ
Tel: 01202 390 008
Fax: 01202 393 621

www.medline.co.uk

The School of Meditation
158 Holland Park Avenue
London W11
Tel: 0171 603 6116

Yoga for Health Foundation Residential Centre
Ickwell Bury
Northill
nr Biggleswade
Bedfordshire SG218 9EF
Tel: 01767 627271

Organic food

Henry Doubleday Research Association
National Centre for Organic Farming
Ryton-on-Dunsmore
Coventry, CV8 3LG

Kjaers Food for Life
56E Upper Montagu Street
London W1H 1FP
Tel: 0171 723 0091

Mail order service includes organic sprouted rye bread and other baked products for special diets.

The Organic Directory
Green Earth Books
Green Books
foxhole
Dartington
Totnes
Devon TQ9 6EB
Tel: 01803 863260

Guide to buying natural foods, including box schemes, covering England, Scotland, Wales and the Channel Island.

The Real Meat Company
Warminster BA12 7BZ
Tel: 01985 840436

The Soil Association Ltd
86–88 Colston Street
Bristol BS1 5BB

Publications include: Directory of Farms shops and Box Schemes, Regional Guide to Buying Organic Food.

The Village Bakery Melmerby
Penrith
Cumbria CA1D 1HE
Tel: 01768 881515

Apart from local availablilty in some supermarkets and health food shops, there is a postal service for this range of baked foods, suitable for people with food sensitivities

Working Weekends on Organic Farms (WWOOF)
19 Bradford Road
Lewes
Sussex BN7 1RB

Opportunities to work part-time on organic farms in return for free accomodation and food.

Supplements and mail order

BioCare
Lakeside
180 Lifford Lane
Kings Norton
Birmingham
B30 3NT
Tel: 0121 433 3929
Fax: 0121 459 4167

Specialist in quality supplements for candida and ME. Their products are also avilable in selected health food shops and specialist pharmacies.

BioCare Denne Pharmacy
North Heath Lane
Horsham RH12 4PJ
Tel: 01403 253943

Nutri Centre
7 Park Crescent
London W1N 3HE
Tel: 0171 436 5122

Also stocks a wide range of books from America.

Nutri Limited
Buxton Road
New Mills
High Peak SK22 3JU
Tel: 0800 212742

Good range of candida supplements.

Nutriscene
Medway Clinic of Nutritional and Bioenergetic Medicine
28 The Precinct
Rainham
Kent ME8 7H
Tel: 01634 362267
Sheridan Stock's own herbal formulations of anti-fungal supplements.

The Pure H20 Company
5 Egham Busness Park
Crabtree Road
Egham
Surrey TW20 8RD
Tel: 0207 681 8241
www.pureh20.co.uk

This system combines gentle reverse osmosis with deionisation to produce pure water, free of disease-causing micro-organisms. Although costly to instal, the system can be rented at a cost which is cheaper than buying water in the supermarket, or delivered to your door.

Revital
85 High Rd
Willesden
London NW19 2TE
Free order number: 0800 252 875

Journals and magazines

Berrydales Special Diet News
Berrydales Publishers
Berrydale House
5 Lawn Road
London NW3 2XS

BioMED Newsletters
16 Court Oak Grove
Harborne
Birmingham B32 2HR

The Inside Story
Useful publication for those with food intolerances, with research information, food tastings, and articles on alternative foods.

What Doctors Don't Tell You
77 Grosvenor Avenue
London N5 2NN
Tel: 020 7354 4592

A lively and informative publication on what doctors don't tell you!

Key words and recipe index